Cutthroat

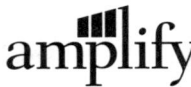

www.amplifypublishing.com

Cutthroat: A Surgeon's Fight against Big Government, Corrupt Businessmen, and a Broken Healthcare System

©2022 Steven J. Cyr. All Rights Reserved. No part of this publication may be reproduced, stored in a retrieval system, or transmitted in any form by any means electronic, mechanical, or photocopying, recording or otherwise without the permission of the author.

For more information, please contact:
Amplify Publishing, an imprint of Mascot Books
620 Herndon Parkway, Suite 320
Herndon, VA 20170
info@amplifypublishing.com

Library of Congress Control Number: 2021923888

CPSIA Code: PRV0122A

ISBN-13: 978-1-63755-304-6

Printed in the United States

For LeAnn, my soulmate—your loving support, intelligence, strength, and encouragement are unparalleled. I'm blessed to have you by my side— through thick and thin.

Cutthroat

A Surgeon's Fight against Big Government, Corrupt Businessmen, and a Broken Healthcare System

STEVEN J. CYR, MD

with **GLENN PLASKIN**

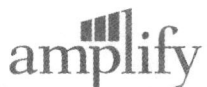

Contents

Introduction 1

CHAPTER 1	Targeted	13
CHAPTER 2	Calm in the Storm	21
CHAPTER 3	My Calling to Medicine	33
CHAPTER 4	Unanswered Prayers	43
CHAPTER 5	A Cinderella Story	61
CHAPTER 6	Surgical Precision	71
CHAPTER 7	The Hornet's Nest	83
CHAPTER 8	Workers' *De*compensation	99
CHAPTER 9	The Love of Money	115
CHAPTER 10	Free at Last	133
CHAPTER 11	"Cutter"	149
CHAPTER 12	To Lease or Not to Lease	163
CHAPTER 13	Et Tu	179
CHAPTER 14	As Sure as the Pope Is Catholic	189
CHAPTER 15	In God We "Trust"	203
CHAPTER 16	Out of the Frying Pan, into the Oven	217
CHAPTER 17	Vindication	227
CHAPTER 18	Beauty from Ashes	241
CHAPTER 19	Pawns and Cons	247

Acknowledgments 263

Source Material 273

Introduction

There isn't anyone on the planet who doesn't deserve excellent healthcare. It's a basic human need. Yet millions of people are either entirely neglected or unsatisfied with the medical attention they're getting.

In fact, among all industrialized nations, the United States has the highest *dissatisfaction* rate when it comes to healthcare. A whopping 79 percent of the population is turned off by a system meant to protect them. High costs, endless red tape, gaping holes in coverage, and poor access are among a handful of reasons. But that's just the beginning.

As a surgeon in practice for the past eighteen years, I've been astounded by the wreckage of our healthcare system, the control given to insurance companies, and the corruption surrounding both doctors and patients. It's a medical jungle with perils lurking everywhere.

Although everyone knows something is wrong, I don't think people actually understand what is happening in American healthcare. Pompous politicians in Washington think they know what's best for us and have passed laws that have had disastrous results for physicians and their patients. Meanwhile, the general public assumes that doctors are rich and that they have control over the care they can provide a patient. But as you'll see, our care is being rationed by insurance companies, and doctors are struggling—as if we were living in a dictatorial country. When it comes to healthcare, we are.

In the pages ahead, you're going to see just how bad it is and who is *really* responsible.

This book is a cautionary tale, one that will shine a bright light on the harsh realities of the medical world as it is today. Things will never change until we are aware of the problem and willing to do something about it.

I believe in standing up for what is right. And I want to expose conditions in our healthcare system that need an overhaul. Trust me, nothing could be more life-altering than the medical care you're *getting* and the conditions under which physicians are *giving* it.

I can tell you that the pressures that accompany the life of a physician are largely unknown. For my fellow practitioners: I hope this book serves as a warning to help you avoid the cutthroat businessmen who surround our profession—the predators who are waiting to devour us, like voracious lions, using whatever means possible. I'm referring not only to medical-industry politics and health-insurance systems that penalize doctors instead of rewarding them but also to people (attorneys and investigators) using the legal systems—both civil and criminal—to mercilessly attack innocent bystanders (i.e., physicians).

These battles—fought behind the scenes as doctors and surgeons endeavor to deliver premier care to patients—have taken an emotional toll on many of us. They steal a large portion of the joy we should feel as healers. All the administrative red tape is draining and expensive, limiting what we can do to attend to the only thing that matters—our *patients*.

And in that sense, I am running out of *patience*, which is why I'm writing this book highlighting my own personal saga of intrigue and manipulation that I hope no other doctor will ever have to endure.

As I've discovered, there are many factions manipulating the landscape of American healthcare for the bottom line. Doctors have been caught in the crosshairs as strong advocates for their patients but weak advocates for themselves. I hesitated in writing this book because I was not sure I wanted to air my "dirty laundry" or suffer any backlash from my revelations. But I decided it was a story that had to be told in order to protect my colleagues from similar experiences and to bring light to the challenges many physicians face.

Beyond this book serving as an exposé for medical insiders attempting to avoid the same circumstances, it also shares a story that may serve anyone who cares about receiving quality healthcare. In so many cases, it's the insurance companies and their lackeys who are holding our nation's doctors hostage, dictating to them what procedures they can and cannot perform. Those companies are able to actually *practice* medicine through multiple tactics, including the peer-to-peer review process. This loophole allows insurance companies to hire peer-review doctors who often are not peers at all (they are often non-surgeons or doctors from a different specialty altogether) and who have never seen the patient to approve or deny care for that specific person. It's a slick way to ration care.

All they do is follow a cookbook recipe of what is approved and what isn't. Whether it's something as minimal as ordering labs and MRI studies or as major as granting approval for a surgery, *they are in control*. They are not considering the patient's well-being. They haven't heard of their sufferings, their illnesses, or their injuries. They don't know the patients. They don't care for or about the patients. They only care about their profits, and there are no negative repercussions to their denials. It is the ultimate conflict of interest. They deny care. They make more money.

I believe no one should interfere with a physician's patient care under the guise of a "peer-to-peer review" or any other financially driven agenda. The final decision for care should be left to the treating doctor and patient—*not* the insurance company, nor even another physician who has not established a doctor–patient relationship. So, in my view, the opinion of the peer-review doctor is *irrelevant*. It's the treating doctor whose medical license is on the line who should direct and determine care. Certainly, whether the medical outcome or surgical result is good or bad, the liability falls to the treating physician and no one else.

Years ago, while I was performing peer reviews for spine-surgery care, I realized the process was not really an effort of the carriers to provide proper care but instead to ration or deny care altogether. After performing these reviews for about two years, the insurance carriers requested the company that hired me no longer use me as a reviewer. Was there a problem with my credentials or my level of knowledge? Did my opinions lead to poor outcomes? Of course not. It had and has nothing to do with looking for correct decision-making and everything to do with the carriers not paying for care.

Apparently, I had authorized the requested treatment and surgery too often. I felt that it wasn't my place to tell doctors how to care for their own patients. So unless I felt the plan would lead to a poor outcome or was dangerous, I would approve treatment as requested. Clearly the goal of the insurance carriers is to deny care, so they only hire doctors and companies who routinely deny treatment. It is a ploy to limit patient care, and it undermines the ability of a doctor to provide adequate treatment to their patients while eliminating the risk for the intervening peer-review doctors and the insurance companies who are essentially practicing medicine.

The shocking truth is that this corporate practice of medicine has violated the power of doctors and the rights of patients; this biased peer-review process and other insidious tactics ensure maximal profits for insurance carriers without much regard for patient health. Imagine: needed surgeries requested by *surgeons* are sometimes initially denied by registered nurses! And they do it under the guise of efficiency and ethics of care. In my opinion, this is only one of many schemes employed to keep the premiums paid by patients for their medical care as profits for the insurance carrier. However, there are many others—and the insurance companies are not the only entities responsible for the challenges we all face in healthcare, as you will read.

I believe insurance carriers and many of the business entities in medicine are often driven by the bottom line, not by what is necessarily good for the patient. And because the insurance carriers are forever whittling away what procedures or interventions they will approve (not to mention issuing paltry physician reimbursements), some doctors feel compelled to cram in as many patient visits and surgeries as possible, all at the expense of quality patient care.

Overall, the media, business world, insurance companies, and even the government have done an amazing job of portraying doctors as the culprits for the exorbitant costs in healthcare. They've been able to make the public believe that all doctors are opportunistic millionaires who prey on the injuries and diagnoses of patients in order to make themselves rich. The delusion is that doctors order unnecessary tests, perform unnecessary surgeries, prescribe too many medications—including narcotics—and charge too much for their services. Meanwhile, large hospital systems charge far more for the same services delivered by their physicians and their ancillary services.

Not all doctors will be able to relate to my story. Many are academic physicians or physicians employed by hospital systems or a large group practice who are likely dealing with different issues, including a lack of control in the delivery of care and administrative tyranny. It is the private independent practitioners, particularly solo specialists, who have been hit the hardest by these tactics.

As an independent practitioner, despite my focus on innovation and patient care rather than profitability, I have faced intense criticism and scrutiny. In an effort to deliver care with academic standards—spending quality time examining and educating my patients—I see far fewer patients than many surgeons. I perform fewer surgeries in a day than most. It's that approach, however, that has ensured outcomes I am very proud of and a surgical success rate rarely seen in my specialty. To improve the delivery of care, and in an attempt to have a say in how care is delivered to my patients, I have invested in businesses that deliver that care.

Being entrepreneurial is not frowned upon in any other business—definitely not to the degree it is in medicine. And it shouldn't be denigrated in medicine either. Financially successful doctors are often assumed to be greedy or unethical, even by fellow physicians. In fact, doctors who are business-minded have the potential to make medicine efficient and even more affordable, if only they had more control. Physician services and ancillary services, such as imaging facilities, urgent care centers, clinical laboratories, cardiac catheterization facilities, and even surgical facilities, often charge far less than large hospital systems delivering the same services.

Most people don't realize that doctors working in the insurance-based medicine world are often not raking in big dollars for their expertise or effort. In most cases, that could not be further from the truth. Most of the doctors I know nowadays are earning low- or mid-level six-figure incomes and working eighty to one hundred hours a week doing lifesaving surgeries and interventions—and even if they are earning more, they are certainly earning it. Doctors are often blamed as the source of ever-increasing healthcare costs, despite the facts that the median pay of a healthcare CEO was more than $9 million, and thirty CEOs made more than $30 million in 2020. The CEOs of the top six health insurance carriers made a combined $236 million in 2020—45 percent more than 2019. Meanwhile, orthopaedic surgery reimbursements fell an average of 28 percent between 1992 and 2007. Doctors saw a 22 percent cut to their reimbursements between 2001 and 2022 and a proposed 9.75 percent cut in 2022 despite the extreme toll the COVID-19 pandemic placed on them mentally and financially. In the same time frame, the cost to run a medical practice has increased 39 percent.

By the time physicians pay their student loans and their practice overhead, there's very little left! Also, considering the workload that doctors endure—as well as the life-changing nature of their work—whatever compensation they earn is certainly justifiable.

I know it's hard for some to believe that doctors can be victims of the system, but they are, just as patients are. We fight every day to prevent the rationing of care that maximizes profits for the business side of medicine, which ultimately has a negative impact on patient care. Good doctors are frustrated by the current plethora of red tape and bureaucratic insurance constrictions. In fact, many of my medical colleagues, if not most, are talking their children out of seeking a career in medicine.

In 2021, Medscape reported that 89 percent of physicians are depressed. Moreover, out of all professions with the highest suicide rates, medical doctors are rated number one due to a variety of factors, including long hours, demanding patients, malpractice lawsuits, medical school debt, and ease of access to medications.

Those are sobering statistics that should give pause to anyone interested in a career in medicine and also to their patients. To make matters worse, many of us are now being investigated and convicted of federal crimes, like common criminals. How did this happen? Who is to blame? And what is the solution?

Like many others, I am not a physician who entered private practice looking to make the "big bucks," although I do believe a person should be paid a fair salary to compensate for their investment in training and knowledge and impact on society. The general public assumes all doctors are multimillionaires, though many of us struggle to pay our bills. We are being crushed by the burden of student loans, practice overhead, forever dwindling reimbursements, and the bureaucratic nightmare of modern American medicine and its tyrannical stranglehold on doctors and patients.

In my case, all my professional goals were slanted toward service, not profit. That's one reason I spent fourteen years serving in the military as a U.S. Air Force physician (not a money-making decision) rather than racing into a more "lucrative" private practice.

I was motivated to serve as a patriot: someone who loves his country. I chose a career in medicine because it was a job that innately required a perspective of self-sacrifice and devotion to others. I have led a life of integrity as an officer in the military and as a man of strong Christian faith. Money has never been my driving force, only service.

But, when I began practicing outside of the military, I realized medicine wasn't what I had envisioned it to be. The reimbursements were controlled and constantly decreased by insurance carriers and the government. Paying overhead was a struggle, and I was soon "pounced" upon by those metaphorical lions—unscrupulous businesspeople who viewed me as "an opportunity." To them, I was a dollar sign, a skilled surgeon on whom they could capitalize in order to generate money for themselves.

In order to protect myself, I tried to navigate the course of my career cautiously, always relying on a certified healthcare attorney to guide my decisions about which offers to consider and which ones to avoid in my effort to have a profitable practice. Like most physicians who are not businessmen, I was susceptible to falling into these legal and financial traps as easily as anyone else. I was raised to be sensible and hardworking and diligent as well as moral and honest. I was brought up in a military family, and I later watched my parents build a successful business. I learned from that example that a hardworking entrepreneur could enjoy more success, freedom, and satisfaction than someone who is traditionally employed. I learned the rules, realized when to ask questions, and had the appropriate advice of my attorneys to guide me. But as you'll see, that advice wasn't always protective.

I hope that all the trials I faced will be a wake-up call to everyone in medicine, including patients who expect their physicians to be at the top of their game and happy in their chosen profession. As I always tell residents and younger colleagues—physicians beware! It is a dangerous game out here. We are *not* adequately equipped to deal with the many business- and insurance-related challenges that surround us as we graduate and begin to practice.

Throughout this book you will see personal examples of several key issues to understand and pitfalls to avoid, including the following:

- Investing in businesses outside your practice
- In-network vs. out-of-network rules and restrictions
- The problem with workers' compensation
- Marketing and consulting agreements
- Leases with personal guarantees
- Avoiding bankruptcy
- Compliance with Stark, Anti-Kickback, and now Racketeer Influenced and Corrupt Organizations (RICO) laws

And for those of you who are *not* practitioners of medicine, I hope that you read this story with empathy, seeing physicians in a new light and understanding the complex pressures and challenges we face. Our life's mission is to ensure that you and your loved ones receive excellent medical care. Most physicians are patient advocates and continue to carry the weight of this responsibility with honor. But we have lost control of medicine; and the strain is becoming unbearable.

   I pray that the experiences you read about here will help guide and protect you in your own life's journey, especially if you are a physician. While this book is intended to shed light on the potential pitfalls for entrepreneurial private practitioners, it is also intended to help anyone in any profession avoid the mistakes I made, whether in medicine, business, or life. Hopefully my experience in the medical world will shed light on the many crucial issues and decisions that all physicians need to understand in order to avoid a life of financial and legal misery. I wish I had been better prepared for it.

Chapter One

Targeted

San Antonio, Texas

I had just completed a fifteen-hour spine surgery. My patient, a sweet sixty-two-year-old grandmother, had spent the last year and a half sleeping upright in a chair. Her spine had collapsed forward at a 90-degree angle—the product of seven failed surgeries performed by five different surgeons.

Tragically, the screws in her spine had penetrated her skin and were now visible from the outside. She was in an obviously desperate state. The surgery I performed was ultimately lifesaving, as the patient had been given only six months to live due to the fluid surrounding her heart and filling her lungs. This fluid retention was a by-product of her inability to inhale deeply or to sit upright.

Since I was a Mayo Clinic–trained spine surgeon with a specialty in correcting failed surgeries and complicated spinal conditions, her family sought my assistance because no one else, including her previous surgeons, was willing to tackle her complicated issue. Her surgery was risky and could have resulted in paralysis or even death. But this surgery was her only hope. As I told her and her family, the recovery would be a long and difficult one. But the surgery, her third procedure over the course of two weeks, was a success: I was able to address her infection, remove her failed hardware (screws and rods), remove and replace her broken/collapsed spinal bones with an expandable metallic cage, and stabilize and straighten her spine with a totally new construct of screws and rods from the top to the bottom of her spine.*

I was excited to see the change the surgery would bring to her life. During the time I was treating her, I had become very strongly connected to her three children. I loved the passion and commitment that all had in seeking help for their mother. I spend a lot of time with my patients, hearing their stories and empathizing with their trials. Sometimes I can truly feel their pain.

In this case, I could feel all three of her adult children's desperation for me to save their mother. They were tearful each time we spoke of her pain and the misery she had experienced over the preceding fifteen years of failed surgery after failed surgery. With each surgery, her function declined further, leaving her in state of constant and unremitting pain. She missed many celebrations, weddings, and family events. She was confined to a chair, could not lie in a bed, and was unable to even walk or stand for any significant length of time.

This was why I became a spine surgeon. I never backed down from a challenging case, despite the risk I assumed. These cases, as

---

* This type of surgery isn't common for most spine surgeons, but it had become commonplace for me secondary to my Mayo training and military background.

challenging as they were for me, were the ones I remember most because the life change that was possible was worth the effort and personal sacrifice. I missed many meals, birthday celebrations, and special events of my own while tackling these difficult surgeries, but I felt obligated out of service to others and a calling from God to make the biggest impact possible in this life.

After I scrubbed out of surgery, fatigued from the physical and mental strain of such a taxing procedure, I looked at my many text messages for any important updates, then I opened my email to review the messages from the day. My eye immediately caught the name of a criminal defense attorney who had represented me years before. Four years prior, a company I had been designing implants for was federally indicted for their business dealings with a U.S. Army surgeon. My records were reviewed, but I was absolved of any wrongdoing and given a release by the federal attorney assigned to that case.

When I left the operating room, I opened the email to see what it said; my heart stopped. The email turned my optimism from the successful surgery to immediate shock and panic: *You are being targeted for federal indictment, and due to a conflict of interest, I can no longer represent you.*

I was in shock, but I still had to compose myself to talk to the family about the surgery. As a surgeon, I had to put my own issues on the back burner. I couldn't let my personal dilemma affect my communication with the family. So I gathered the X-rays and collected my thoughts. I approached the family calmly, and I explained we were able to accomplish everything we set out to and that their mother was stable.

When I left the waiting room, I looked back at my phone to re-read the email. I couldn't believe what I was reading. *What in the world was going on?!* I had no idea what he was talking about, but I would soon find out that my wife, LeAnn, did. When I called her, she explained to me that earlier that day, she had read that email and subsequently called the attorney. But she had not alerted me to it, because she did not want to alarm me during my operation. She had been in a total panic all day long, waiting for me to get out of surgery.

LeAnn—who is very levelheaded in a crisis—had already contacted an attorney friend who recommended we reach out to Mike McCrum. Mike McCrum was a former federal attorney, a strong Christian, and one of the most respected criminal defense attorneys in San Antonio. He was so well-known that even our daughter, Alexa, who was in the car with LeAnn during the terrifying phone call, knew who he was.

Alexa was impressed when she observed him in a trial while interning with our friend Nico LaHood, the Bexar County district attorney. Fortunately, McCrum was available to represent us and immediately contacted our previous "conflicted" attorney. We had some peace in knowing McCrum was on our side but, as a former Air Force officer who prides himself on his integrity, I was distraught over the idea that I was being targeted.

That night, I sat in my bedroom feeling tormented and vulnerable—more discouraged than I had ever been in my entire life. I had a million questions...but no answers.

Why was I being targeted for federal indictment? Who initiated the allegation to generate an investigation? Why would my previous attorney be conflicted and unable to represent me?

My wife and I sat down, baffled at this vague and ominous message, and tried to decipher what it meant.

At this point in my life, I was at the top of my game: I was a well-respected spine surgeon and a former professor of orthopaedic surgery. Over a period of fourteen years, I had created a highly successful medical practice—one of the top-rated spine clinics in Texas. I had received many top honors for patient care, being rated a top doctor by numerous ratings companies, including Castle Connolly, as well as *Texas Monthly*, America's Top 10, RateMDs, and Vitals.com. I owned a busy practice, The Orthopaedic & Spine Institute (OSI), with twenty-two fellow doctors and mid-level providers and 105 support staff.

I had been the chief of spine surgery for the U.S. Air Force and served two tours of duty in Iraq during Operation Enduring Freedom, receiving a Meritorious Service Medal. I was also the spine surgery consultant to the surgeon general of the U.S. Air Force and the Pentagon.

In short, I had worked hard, and everything seemed to be going my way.

With that email, my world came crashing down. What happened reminds me a little of the movie *Molly's Game*, about a former Olympic-class skier who ran the world's most exclusive high-stakes poker game and ultimately became an FBI target. But this wasn't a movie; and the protagonist wasn't some stranger or a potential criminal—*it was me*. I was a physician taking care of patients, not running an underground gambling ring.

I was no gambler...at least I didn't think I was. Little did I realize at the time, I had gambled my entire future by unknowingly aligning myself with unscrupulous business partners. Several of my business affiliations ended up disastrous; they were almost career-ending. The safe world I thought I had created for myself, my wife, LeAnn, and our four children imploded.

In a flash, I was not only betrayed by physicians in my practice, but I was also used as a scapegoat by a business partner who attempted to entangle me in his web of perpetual lies when he was indicted for healthcare fraud and marijuana trafficking.

I was investigated by the FBI and the U.S. Department of Labor, the subject of a grueling two-year probe. Agents sifted through ten years of our financial records, emails, and corporate documents, and they questioned more than 350 people in the medical field about me.

To make matters worse, I would also become the target of two separate billion-dollar corporations that accused me of fraud, attempting to take everything we owned, including our home.

All this turmoil began with that email, but the attacks just kept coming. I lost the hospital I had founded with all the savings I had worked so hard to earn by practicing seven days per week for years on end. I was forced to close my medical practice, and I was even driven into bankruptcy court.

And of course, I could easily have lost my medical license too. Thankfully, due to my innocence, I did not.

Not least harmful, I was dragged through the media with headlines that almost ruined my reputation. My family and I were the subjects of a malicious *Forbes* article written by a self-serving bankruptcy attorney who twisted the facts—impugning me and my family, misrepresenting the truth, and drawing flawed conclusions about our guilt. His aspersions, as you'll read, infuriated my wife, LeAnn, who began a campaign to fight back and to protect our privacy and our children. Although she showed immeasurable strength, it wasn't an easy time for us.

As I look back on it now, I often ask myself, *How did a military kid and former decorated lieutenant colonel in the U.S. Air Force who had followed every rule—never broken a law; never drank, smoked, nor tried a drug—end up being the subject of these attacks and a scandalous write-up in a national business magazine?* I had checked off every box when it came to medical integrity. I had sought and *followed* legal advice for every move I made.

And yet there I was. It all began with my being drawn into one of the biggest healthcare scandals in modern history, although I had nothing to do with the hospital, administrators, or doctors being indicted.

It was astonishing to think that doctors and administrators from Dallas were being indicted for violating conflict-of-interest laws for healthcare fraud and that somehow it had spilled over into my world. According to the *Dallas Morning News*, a group of nine was being accused of violating Racketeer Influenced and Corrupt Organizations (RICO) laws, which had first been passed by Attorney General Robert F. Kennedy in the 1960s to convict the mafia. *Yes, the mafia!* I've been told that this law is rarely, if ever, applied to doctors treating patients, but in any event, I certainly had not violated it! I hadn't broken *any* of the rules. Though I was innocent, I was treated as if I was guilty. My name was slandered by investigators throughout San Antonio and Houston, where I practiced.

How could this reversal of fortune have happened? Who could've ever expected it? What was happening in medicine to expose physicians to this type of legal risk and stress—factors that compounded the pressure of having a patient's life in their hands?

Let's just say that I felt like I was being attacked from every angle. Doctors know that medicine can be cutthroat, beginning with the stiff academic competition in college to gain entrance into medical school; then in medical school, as we fight to get into prestigious residency programs; and continuing through residency and even fellowship training. We also know our colleagues can be mercenary in academic and private practice, all vying for recognition as a top physician or surgeon. But this legal attack was a whole new level with much higher stakes, including federal criminal-law implications that I never expected to face as a physician. It reminded me of the times I was deployed to Iraq, under the constant risk of incoming artillery. But this time it wasn't mortars that were threatening my life. Instead, it was a combination of fatalistic factors that obliterated my medical practice, tarnished my public standing, and threatened my ability to survive professionally and financially.

My story is relevant *not* because it's about me. I am just one of many physicians working in the trenches within a broken American healthcare system; I am impacted by it just as many other honest physicians are. It's relevant because physicians are tired, unhappy, and depressed with the state of medicine in America. Many physicians, especially surgeons, feel attacked, overwhelmed, and underappreciated. We feel surrounded and powerless to do what is necessary for our patients, and no one seems to know or care. This is how it all began...

Chapter Two

Calm in the Storm

In the life-and-death world of a surgeon, you have to be laser-focused and able to shut out all distractions around you to concentrate solely on your patient. With a life literally in your hands, it's the highest-stakes game imaginable, with no room for error. You not only need a steady hand but an equally calm inner core, which allows you to *operate* no matter what. This means that even if bombs are exploding around you—which happened to me when I served in the Air Force as a battlefield physician in Iraq—you can't lose a beat. And I never did—even though what I saw from the field shocked me.

It was nonstop horror, with bodies blown up and burned. It was absolutely horrendous. Yet my team and I successfully performed more than seven hundred surgeries under these life-threatening conditions. All the panic around us had to be blocked out. Although my safety was often threatened, I didn't feel afraid. I never wavered in my wartime responsibilities. I couldn't.

Reflecting on it now, I believe my upbringing (with a father who had a volatile temper) had a positive impact on my ability to shut out emotional chaos. Though Dad was sometimes out of control emotionally, I learned to contain my feelings and never lose control. This inner resolve was branded into me right from the start. That skill, honed because I was raised by an emotionally labile father, served me well throughout my life. This skill allows me to maintain my composure—whether that be while enduring physical, professional, or legal challenges. It allows me to compartmentalize my own struggles while I focus on my patients and their issues. It ensures that, no matter how bad things seem to be going, I never arrive home angry or frustrated to the point that I take it out on the people around me.

On the outside, I don't think many people realize the turmoil I sometimes have to keep at bay. I have my dad to thank for that.

I was a military brat who spent my entire life living on Air Force bases in government housing, bouncing from the Philippines to Florida, from Alabama to Texas, observing military culture up close; it is a long family tradition. My paternal grandfather, Merle Cyr, was a cook in the Army. My dad, Kenneth, was a medic and a physician assistant in the Air Force. As the third-generation Cyr, I would one day rise to becoming a lieutenant colonel in the Air Force, the chief orthopaedic spine surgeon for the entire service.

Like any kid who migrates from place to place, I became highly adaptable. You learn the art of fitting in. Even when you feel like the new kid in class, you persevere and adapt to different schools and cultures. No doubt, that's how I absorbed the straight-ahead sense of protocol and self-control that drove me forward my entire life. Ironically, I can see now that it was my father's complicated personality that ultimately prepared me to remain resolutely calm no matter what.

My parents' love story had not been a smooth one. It was a little like the pauper and the princess. When they first met at Clark Air Base in the Philippines, Kenneth Cyr was just a poor twenty-year-old American GI who had gone straight into the Air Force from high school, hoping to capitalize on the educational opportunities the military provided.

Raised in a working-class family in the Carolinas, my dad had a brilliant scientific mind and a real thirst for knowledge. While he had desperately wanted to be a veterinarian, his family didn't have the financial resources to put him through college. Instead, he served during the Vietnam War as an airman, the lowest enlisted rank in the U.S. Air Force.

Meanwhile, my mother, Maria Centenera, was a Spanish–Filipino aristocrat, the third eldest of four girls with a single mother whose husband had died years prior. The illustrious family was well known in the Philippines, having been given land grants by King Philip. In fact, my mother's paternal grandmother was actually a Spanish countess with a father who had owned large tracts of land that spanned from one mountain range to the next.

By the time my dad met my mom, her family firmly opposed the idea of a romance between the simple airman and their precious daughter, but they underestimated my dad's perseverance. He was respectful and soft-spoken, but he laid it all on the line to capture my mother's heart.

My mother was a striking beauty; she was tall by Filipino standards at five foot seven with long auburn hair and an air of refinement about her, thanks to years of formal etiquette training. She was an actress, model, and college student who could have chosen any partner from a leading family. So, considering her pedigree and exquisitely elegant manners, how could she have chosen the rough American who had never even gone to college? On the surface, it seemed like a mismatch, but my father was nothing if not determined.

He was enamored with her beauty and even her air of superiority. She stood out from the rest of the women he had met. She was educated, dignified, and seemed uninterested and unavailable. He was a talented guitarist and had a great voice, so he would sing to her in an attempt to woo her. When he was relaxed, my father was appealing because he had a quiet confidence and bright blue eyes and was extremely articulate and clearly intelligent. My mother began to take notice. He was also not willing to give up easily. He showered her with flowers, was a gentleman, and protected her from disrespectful locals at times. He once described an encounter in which a local Filipino touched my mother's bottom as she entered a public-transport vehicle. My mother slapped him, which resulted in the man rearing his hand back to punch. My father promptly stuck the tip of his umbrella in the man's throat and suggested he leave the vehicle before he got hurt. The man complied. My father wasn't a big guy, but he was not afraid. I'm sure those little things eventually revealed his sincerity and devotion.

After a short courtship of only a few weeks, he was in love and just *knew* he wanted to marry my mother. He needed to do it quickly, because he was planning to separate from the Air Force and return to South Carolina to begin nursing school. He courted her in traditional Spanish–Filipino custom. When he met her family, he showed appropriate deference and respect, and when he felt compelled to propose, he asked her mother and eldest sister (since her father had passed away) for permission to marry her beforehand.

As the family story goes, he told my mother, "If you don't want to marry me, then I'm going to put myself on *international hold*," a status that would embroil my father in legal dispute, thus delaying his return to the United States and allowing him more time to court my mother. My mom thought, *Wow, this guy must really be sincere if he's willing to get himself in trouble just so we can stay together.*

The ploy worked. My mother married my father just two months after they met, but it didn't turn out to be an easy life or a blissful marriage. The naïve romance and high hopes of my parents' brief courtship were replaced by the realities of married life.

Upon returning from the Philippines to Rockhill, South Carolina, in 1967, my dad enrolled full-time in nursing school while my mother had to work her first blue-collar job as a respiratory technician. That same year, my dad's dream of becoming a civilian medical professional was quashed when my mom got pregnant; she gave birth to my older brother Bryan in 1968. This hit the family finances hard, which made it impossible for my dad to continue his full-time nursing education.

Despite my mother's aristocratic background, and all the appearances of wealth, it turned out that she couldn't help him out financially at all. *Her* father had died when she was only seven, so her proud mother had been living for years on an inheritance that had dwindled.

To solve the financial crunch, they decided that my father should re-enter the military and pursue his medical education, which would be entirely paid for by the Air Force. So, in late 1969, Dad re-enlisted and was immediately assigned to Eglin Air Force Base in Florida as a medic; he stayed there until 1971, the year I was born.

What followed were a series of zigzag moves from one military base to another. It wasn't easy on my mom. Once, while Dad spent three months in the Philippines scouting ahead on a new assignment, Mom was forced to temporarily live with her in-laws; we were crowded together in a small home with no heat in the bedrooms, and all of us were huddled under an electric blanket. This was certainly not the life she had envisioned.

We ultimately joined Dad in the Philippines for eighteen months, after which he was accepted into the physician assistant program in Wichita Falls, Texas. Being a PA was a brand-new profession back then, and it allowed him to channel his passion for medicine. However, unlike most servicemen in the Air Force with a bachelor's degree, PAs did not receive a commission as an officer at that time.*

PAs also didn't get the respect that doctors did; back then, doctors were held up on a pedestal, according to my father. He would complain often of how doctors got all the recognition and respect and that PAs were treated poorly. He envied their status. This dichotomy left Dad feeling degraded, like a second-class medical care provider. It was a wound that would never heal. Imagine what it was like for him: he knew he had the intellectual ability to become a physician but had been hindered by family finances, and he couldn't seem to shake it off.

He would live an existence of dissatisfaction and resentment for the majority of his life, always complaining about how he was not viewed with the level of respect he deserved. It was as if his self-esteem had been permanently damaged. Unfortunately, he unleashed his frustration at home. Patience was not his strong suit.

---

*   My dad was actually one of the first Air Force PAs and would later successfully lobby Congress so that physician assistants could be promoted to officers.

More often than not, he was volatile, bullheaded, and aggressive. He had a short fuse and a very loud voice, often losing his temper and shouting at the top of his lungs at me, my brothers, and mother. Anything could set him off. His tantrums, like a tornado, would rip through the entire household.

Though he wasn't home that much due to his responsibilities on base, he made it very clear that *he* was the commander of the household; he was very much a disciplinarian who didn't tolerate disrespect or poor manners. He made sure that we chewed with our mouths closed and kept our elbows off the table. Like most conscientious parents, he watched our every move. But his response to poor manners was extreme and threatening. We learned to be well behaved out of fear, not patient, loving guidance.

"Do it right the first time," he'd say. He was certainly not a warm fuzzy kind of dad. "Get your head out of your goddamn ass!" he'd holler at least a few times a day. At the peak of his outbursts, he would sometimes grab us by both ears and scream directly in our faces. And even though he was an academic, he rarely helped me with my studies or assignments. "Go look it up!" was another one his mottos. This one in particular forced me to become more independent and proactive. His reluctance to "hold my hand" through challenges would serve me later in life by teaching me self-reliance and perseverance. My ability to concentrate despite chaos and even physical threats served me later as a surgeon in a war zone and in civilian life when I needed to focus intently on the surgeries I was performing. While some children may have fallen into the trap of repeating bad behaviors as adults, I was able to filter out only the good behaviors and emulate them.

His erratic mood swings definitely impacted the atmosphere of our household. It seemed as if Dad was frustrated and angry nearly all the time. We were never physically beaten, but his behavior was definitely verbally abusive—especially toward my mother. She was far less emotional than Dad and typically remained restrained in the eye of the storm. No matter what her innermost feelings, she was an elegant and very kind woman who radiated an air of nobility.

However, she suffered, and my brothers and I always felt bad for her. Even as little kids, we knew that my father was wrong, that his temper tantrums were unacceptable. To this day, I wonder why my mother took a chance and married the poor American in the first place. She had been raised in a family that was quiet and classy; they were prideful people who treated one another with respect. She must have been taken aback and disappointed in Dad's behavior. But she stayed with him anyway. No doubt she did it out of love for us, a general sense of loyalty, and because she knew deep down that my father had a kind heart. She knew he had other positive qualities as well, including a strong work ethic.

Another reason she stayed was because she was a devout Catholic and didn't believe in separation or divorce, so she was going to make their marriage work no matter what. Her faithfulness and devotion to my dad really surprised me. I *still* wonder how she was able to tolerate his behavior. But she once told me that, through all her challenges with his personality, "it was more important that you and your brothers had a father in your lives than for me to have the perfect marriage." I'll never forget that sacrifice.

As faithful a woman as she was, and though she struggled with this situation, she learned to deal with it in her own way. Wisely, instead of becoming Dad's adversary or withdrawing, she became kind of a cheerleader. She eventually pushed him to reach his goals academically, as he earned one degree after another.

In fact, though he felt undervalued, he nonetheless stayed put in the Air Force for the next twenty-plus years. Beyond his PA certification, he also got a nursing degree and eventually earned three master's degrees and two PhDs—one in counseling psychology and another in clinical psychology. All this together was impressive and provided needed financial security, as our family of four expanded to five when my youngest brother, Michael, was born in 1980. As Dad rose in rank in the Air Force to major and got more respect, his moods improved slightly.

However, despite his accomplishments, nothing could change his underlying emotional liability. His emotional outbursts were always unpredictable and untimely. He would yell and raise his voice at my mother—even in church. We were all embarrassed by it.

As I mentioned earlier, this motivated me to stay calm and control my own emotions. Rather than mirroring the behavior of my father, I did the exact opposite. Dad had unknowingly taught me the art of restraint and given me the ability to *detach* from conditions around me to maintain my own equilibrium.

And years later, when I became a spine surgeon, the emotional imprint of my childhood served me well. It actually *helped* me function. It's somewhat ironic how my father's lack of control imbued in me the ability to maintain it.

Despite the mood shifts, Dad had a softer, sweet side too. He would wake my mother by wiping her face with a warm washcloth in the mornings. He was also fun and spirited at times. He always made the holidays special. He was artistic and would create homemade Halloween costumes for us all that were very cool. He also decorated the house for Christmas and would stomp up on the roof and ring a bell to simulate reindeer before we received our gifts from Santa. To say he loved the outdoors is an understatement. As a result, he taught us many life skills on adventures throughout the world. My father was somewhat of a Renaissance man. He took us hunting and fishing with him, set our lures, put bait on our hooks, and taught us how to survive off the land and take care of ourselves. He also took care of us when we were sick and taught us to be responsible, take pride in our actions, be honest, work hard, and get an education. But he also played the guitar and sang, was a talented artist and poet, and wrote numerous heartfelt poems about his dreams and experiences. He even had one published in *Chicken Soup for the Nurse's Soul* called "Love in Your Hands," which tells the story of a nurse and a nursing-home patient who was grateful for the loving care he provided. He was definitely more bark than bite, but his bark was pretty loud and scary to a little kid. As I grew up, I could see my father was tormented by his childhood. I later found out that he felt unloved by his mother and resented being unable to go to veterinary school. He was frustrated and angry, but deep down he was a good man. He taught me a lot over the years, but most importantly, I was inspired by Dad's special gift as a healer.

   Throughout my childhood, he always demonstrated a nurturing side that came out when we were injured or sick, taking meticulous care of me and my brothers. His demeanor changed completely in that role. He took tremendous pride in his ability to help and heal. For example—when I broke my arm, he splinted it carefully; when I split my lip open on a coffee table, he sewed it up perfectly. When we were sick, he brought us medicine and checked on us frequently. As time passed, I was always absorbing what he did to heal others in need and *how* he did it.

Sometimes I even visited his clinic and observed how he took care of patients in professional settings. He was amazingly empathic, and he sincerely cared. I learned from him the value of hard work, a devotion to education, and the importance of service to others. I could observe that he had a genuinely kind heart, together with all the qualities that made him a superb clinician, and it was this devotion to medicine that intrigued me.

Even at the age of four, I remember thinking that I was going to go into the medical profession. At first, I wanted to be a dentist. But by age eight, I'd decided to become a physician. I loved the idea of being able to help people who were hurt or sick, and this career choice was totally aligned with my mother's point of view.

In her mind—as was typical in Spanish–Filipino culture—there were only two credible jobs in the world: you either became a doctor or a lawyer. That was it. My mother's wish was that I pursue medicine. I felt as if I *had* to excel in order to gain her respect. Motivated by my natural inclination for medicine and my mother's perspective, I did everything I could to set myself up academically. I became a devoted and diligent student with excellent grades, so that I could one day go to medical school.

I was also athletic as a kid and excelled in basketball, football, and martial arts. My earliest days were spent on Eglin Air Force Base in Fort Walton Beach, Florida, a 464,000-acre compound adjacent to the Gulf of Mexico—truly a mammoth "backyard" for a kid. Thereafter, we completed two tours in the Philippines, the second of which started at age eleven and lasted until I was nearly finished with high school.

There we were, three brothers—all born in different places and all us on the move as military brats, circling the globe before my memory of it all could even kick in. It was a blur.

No matter where we lived, I was always wanting to be outside playing any sport I could. But my parents weren't sports fans at all. They were all about academic excellence, and they drilled into me the idea that excelling in school would ensure my future success in life. I definitely got the message, but I thrived on the football field as well.

I listened to their many lessons, and I did want to be a physician, but I wasn't about to give up on my goal of becoming a professional football player too. I learned to balance that dream with academics. I knew success in either field would take dedication and perseverance, but I was pretty driven. I had no doubt I would achieve those goals. I soaked in all the advice my parents gave me. Their lofty expectations and academic demands fueled my passion to excel. All of my childhood experiences, both the good and the bad, molded me into someone with tremendous resolve and the ability to handle pressure, stress, noise, and even chaos while remaining calm and collected. These gifts would serve me well in the years to come.

Chapter Three

My Calling to Medicine

By the time I was eleven, we had moved back to the Philippines, which is where I stayed until I was seventeen. Of any of the places we ever lived, I loved living on Clark Air Base the most. Being in my mother's homeland, I *felt* the power of family warmth for the first time in my life. Among our Spanish and Filipino relatives, I had so many aunts, uncles, and cousins who were gracious and hospitable—some prosperous and some not. As for us, we always lived in military housing, which only improved a bit in size as my father rose through the ranks to an officer. But it really didn't matter. I just loved being in the Philippines, surrounded by all the families and kids with the structure of a close-knit community around me. In fact, the entire experience of living in a foreign culture formed the way I think about life, and it led to unexpectedly meeting people who would change the course of my life.

First off, being the foreigner in a developing nation makes you appreciate the conveniences and the comforts of America because you don't *have* them anymore. Life for many in the Philippines is quite tough. As an impressionable eleven-year-old, I was shocked by the level of poverty and financial struggle around me; it was unlike anything I had ever seen.

I could understand why Filipinos idolized the American lifestyle and wanted to escape their country to come to America. It would break your heart to see children as young as four years old begging in the street without shoes or pants. Often their clothes would be soiled and tattered. Young women from all over the country would flock to the areas surrounding the military bases, selling their bodies in hope of marrying an American GI to break their cycle of poverty.

There were squatters who would build shanty homes on private property with just a few square feet of land to occupy. Makeshift cardboard boxes would become home to the poorest of the poor. During the hurricane monsoon season, these fragile cardboard dwellings and ramshackle huts would wash away in the floods. To say the least, conditions were tragic for many, which made me always appreciate our secure life on a military base and the benefits that came with being an American.

In fact, unlike most kids in conventional schools back in the United States, my experience as a military brat made me understand the sacrifices that service members make to serve and defend our country. At school, we didn't just say the Pledge of Allegiance. I saw patriotism up close on a daily basis, and I understood what our military was doing and why. I was taking all this in. I might never have become an Air Force surgeon had I not grown up living on a military base in the first place.

As a foreigner in a developing nation, I was thrown into a culture that made me appreciative of all races and cultures. It was a melting pot with total mutual acceptance. Ethnicities had nothing to do with our choice of relationships and alliances. In fact, all the kids I met bonded together, becoming much closer than you typically see in schools in America.

Many of us were children of foreign mothers; others were from all regions of the United States. It was truly a cool blend of disparate ethnicities and backgrounds all coming together in one congenial place. As I think back on it now, being thrown into a culture like this was an invaluable experience that later enhanced my ability to a navigate in the world as an adult, allowing me to relate to all types of people and circumstances.

Aside from my academic abilities and aspiration to become a doctor, I excelled at two other things in school that I loved—football and breaking (breakdancing)! Yes, back in the eighties, my older brother Bryan and I were "breakers" and "poppers," proud to be in a multiethnic dance crew of six called the Fantastic Force.

Breaking, also called *breakdancing* or *b-boying/b-girling*, is an acrobatic style of street dance with four kinds of movement: top-rock, down-rock, power moves, and freezes. Think about when guys spin on their backs and on their heads and hands. That's breakin'.

Popping is also a street dance, performed standing, that involves quickly contracting and relaxing muscles to cause a jerk or a sudden stop in the dancer's body, referred to as a *pop* or a *hit*. Other forms are moving your arms and body in a smooth wavelike motion called *waving* or stopping abruptly at each joint, called *ticking*.

Michael Jackson's moonwalk is a classic and masterful popping move. A lot of those moves have been incorporated into modern dance, and you'll see early examples of breaking and popping in the movie *Flashdance*. When Jennifer Beals spun on her back and did a windmill, that's a breaking move. The dancer in the movie was actually a good friend of mine and an icon in the breakin' world who wore a wig for the part. His name is Crazy Legs, a pioneer of the now-famous artform originally from the Bronx. Before we were friends, we learned how to break and pop from watching his movies and videos of his crew, the Rock Steady Crew, battling other crews in New York City. As you can tell from my detailed description, dancing was a big deal to me back then.

In fact, breakdancing changed my life in more than one way. It's how I met a beautiful, young girl named LeAnn Bergerud, who would one day become my wife! As I see it now, proximity can truly be the messenger of fate.

When LeAnn and I first met in middle school, I was thirteen and she was twelve. Her American father worked for the Air Force as a civil engineer, and her mother was Vietnamese. We instantly clicked as friends. And as I later found out, she loved watching me break and pop with my buddies. I was the youngest kid in our dance crew, and we won every competition and talent show on or off the base.

I can tell you that breaking was actually my favorite part of growing up in the Philippines—the exhilaration of dancing and winning multiple battles against stiff competition. And because of it, we got popular on and off base really fast. Everybody knew who we were.

Unfortunately, off base, the local dance crews were primarily gangsters, and they hated losing. In the Philippines, it seemed you could do anything that was unethical or illegal without any repercussions. In fact, one of the leaders of a local breaking crew, the Whooze, wanted to kill me and my brother—simply because our group beat them all the time! It also was because our crew was comprised of African Americans, Puerto Ricans, Filipinos, and Caucasian kids. Let's just say that a lot of the locals did not appreciate diversity like we did.

Because we grew up in a third-world country, we were also exposed to a lot of vices: drugs, prostitutes, alcohol, and crime. A lot of kids from the base made the typical bad-teenager decisions and got into drinking and drugs and partying. But I never did. I always stayed away from that stuff. I would go off base just to dance, and then I'd go back on base and make sure I took care of *business*, which was school and weightlifting.

Unfortunately, by the time eighth grade rolled around, just as we were starting to get to know each other better, LeAnn's father got reassigned to a base in Washington, DC, and she moved back to the States. It wasn't until fourteen years later that we would reconnect through a mutual friend and fall in love. Talk about fate. More on that later.

In addition to dancing and martial arts, from the time I was eleven, I was also naturally inclined toward football, playing both running back and linebacker. In fact, I focused almost all of my athletic efforts on football. I loved scoring touchdowns the most. Although I definitely intended to become a doctor, I wanted to play college football *first*. In fact, I imagined playing in the NFL for a couple of years and then going to medical school.

I was confident that I would one day go to the NFL. But, as I said earlier, I got no parental encouragement. Both of my parents were always talking negatively about sports. "You're never going to get anywhere," they'd say. "You're going to *cripple* yourself." They were hyper-focused only on academics, which meant they had little appreciation for my athletic abilities. It was almost as if sports were beneath them. In fact, my father never watched even one of my games; my mother attended very few, and she was confused by the sport, so much so that she didn't even realize that I was *good* at football. She couldn't understand the draw to such a "violent sport." She didn't realize that one learns life values in the trenches while struggling physically alongside others to achieve a common goal. Athletics, particularly team sports, teach us valuable lessons about losing graciously, winning with humility, and the thrill of victory that comes from hours of struggle and toil and even past failures.

Because of this, it was really my big brother, Bryan, who became my biggest supporter in sports. Growing up, Bryan was truly my best friend, and we shared a bedroom until I was sixteen. Ironically, even though he was almost three years older, I always felt very protective of *him*. I had his back and he had mine. We were a pretty adventurous duo. Once we were in our teens, Bryan and I would hop onto available military flights during summers to travel to Air Force bases all over Asia, including Osan Air Base in Korea, Yokota Air Base in Japan, and Kadena Air Base in Okinawa. While in those countries, we traveled to local hot spots off base to learn about the country and its local traditions. We felt so grown up and excited to experience new cultures that few people could ever see.

During the school year, Bryan would come to all my games to cheer me on as only a brother could; he also encouraged me to pursue football in college. I was also immensely supported by one of our high school football coaches, Coach Dogan. On multiple occasions, he'd tell me that I needed to get back to the States so I could get a football scholarship. "You're one of the few athletes here talented enough to play NCAA Division I football," he often told me. I can never forget his confidence in me to pursue my passion in football despite the challenge I would later face as a walk-on.*

Despite my focus on football, I never disappointed my parents when it came to academics. Like my dad, I had a knack for science and math, so nothing distracted me or ever interfered with my academic performance. Even at the peak of the breaking and football season, I worked really hard in school and always made sure I had an A in every class.

I never fell into any of the typical teenage distractions either. I never drank, not one sip of alcohol. I never smoked a cigarette. I never tried any drugs. Instead, I was a very serious and devoted student, always either doing my homework or working out (i.e., lifting weights and practicing martial arts in the off-season from football). Rather disciplined for just a kid, I drove myself academically and physically from the start, never losing focus on my goal of becoming a doctor. Nothing was going to deter me from that goal.

Unfortunately, by the end of high school, I was uprooted yet again; I was forced to move from my beloved Philippines, leaving behind the close friends I had made over a period of seven years. I couldn't believe it. Right in the middle of my senior year, instead of staying to graduate with my friends, I had to suddenly return to the States when my father retired from the Air Force.

This disruption really bothered me. I have no idea why we couldn't have waited a few months for me to finish school. This meant I had to start up at a new high school in San Antonio, Texas. It was disappointing and a real struggle for me. But once again,

---

* In 2020, Coach Dogan contracted COVID-19 and sadly succumbed to the dreaded illness. Our memories of his coaching and constant encouragement live on.

it taught me how to adapt to difficult circumstances and how to persevere and maneuver challenges.

I was initially startled by American culture. After so many years in the Philippines, coming back "home" didn't actually feel familiar at all. It was surreal. I felt like *I* was in a foreign country. In the Philippines, I could just ride my moped to school. But now, even though I was a senior, I took the bus, as we had no money for a car. However, this wasn't the only major adjustment. I was accustomed to only having one American television station. Now we had dozens. I was used to kids from all cultures and financial backgrounds hanging out in the same crowd. I wore a three-finger ring with my breaking nickname, "Baby C," on it and baggy jeans, and I had blow-dried hair with a tall flattop. I definitely stood out. Meanwhile, at my new high school, a lot of the kids wore tight blue jeans, cowboy hats, big belt buckles, and boots. Others dressed more casually, but no one dressed like me...not even remotely.

The funny thing is, because of my unusual appearance, some of the kids who were clearly into drugs thought that I was a narc (an undercover narcotics agent). I guess my attire was so outlandish to them that they assumed I was an adult trying to fit in. In fact, on the assumption that I was an undercover police officer, those guys—who were poster children for the *Just Say No* campaign—planned to jump me! I thought it was funny. They realized it might be a bad idea when I went to the school gym for the first time and bench pressed 375 pounds (which was more than the school football team's maximum)! Even better, Bryan, who knew some of them, confronted some of the dopeheads and told them that I was his brother and not a narc.

Despite this bumpy start, I quickly acclimated, graduating with a class of kids that I only knew for four months. Although there were some amazing people there who welcomed me warmly and I had gone to elementary school with, I would have preferred to graduate with my friends at Clark Air Base. In fact, feeling more isolated than I had in the Philippines, I decided not to go very far from my family when it came to attending college.

Now that we were back in the States, my father took full advantage of the opportunities to hunt and always asked me to accompany him. My father was an avid hunter and fisherman, but he often took it to an extreme. Like most hunters, he would explain that he was only hunting things that he would actually eat and not hunting for "the kill." From the time I was five years old until I was eighteen, we went on many hunting and fishing trips all over the world. However, after a fateful hunting trip with him after we moved back, I realized that aside from our passion for medicine, we were not alike in many other ways.

This trip was during the heat of Texas summer, and we were hunting rabbits. I had never hunted rabbits before and had no idea what I was in for. You see, we weren't hunting those unattractive, gangly jackrabbits. We were out to hunt cottontail rabbits. You know, the ones that are fuzzy, cute, round little balls of fur.

The brush was so thick that it was difficult to move through it. I found myself crawling under it and weaving my body in and out of thorn-covered branches until I would happen upon an unsuspecting rabbit that thought it was protected by the thick brush. When I pulled the trigger of my shotgun, my proximity to the rabbits was so close that it literally blew them away.

After I fired the first shot, I felt uneasy, but I continued the hunt. However, the second rabbit that I shot sealed the deal for me; I knew this wasn't right. The second rabbit ended up getting shot in the gut and hind legs because of the brush surrounding it. I cringed as I noticed it was literally crawling away using his front paws in an attempt to escape me.

The image of that poor little creature crawling away will literally haunt me for the rest of my life. It was in that exact moment that I realized I wasn't meant to be a hunter. I was meant to be a healer. I wasn't put on this earth to take life but instead to improve, and maybe even save, lives.

After that horrific shot, I found my father and explained to him my moral dilemma with tears in my eyes. I told him that I was sorry but that I could not hunt with him ever again. I know that was a hard pill for my father to swallow, because it was literally the only thing we did together. I just didn't have the stomach for it any longer. I loved my father, and for years I had tortured myself on all his crazy excursions to spend time with him, but I just couldn't do it anymore. We both loved excelling academically, but that's where the similarities ended. I didn't get any satisfaction out of hunting. I decided that day that I wasn't going to do things that weren't in sync with who I was as a person to gain anyone's approval, including my father's. He loved hunting and camping and being outdoors. I really enjoyed the comfort of the indoors. I loved sports. He had no interest in sports. In the end, this unfortunate realization meant we would spend little time together from this day forward. I tried for years to bond with him by accompanying him on all kinds of crazy adventures, even though I had no real joy doing so. He chose to never attend my games or performances. Sadly, this difference of interests led to us drifting further apart over the years.

Chapter Four

Unanswered Prayers

As high school was coming to an end, to stay close to my family, I applied to only three nearby schools in Texas; I was offered academic scholarships to all of them, including UT Austin. But instead, I chose to attend Southwest Texas State University (now Texas State University). One of the underlying reasons for going there, much to the chagrin of my parents, was to play football with significantly higher potential of actually making it on the team. Since I never played high school football in the States, I knew my chances of making it on a team like the University of Texas were slim to none. Although academically it was the much stronger school, I couldn't shake my desire to play football. So, I chose Southwest Texas State University over UT—despite a massive four-year scholarship—to play football.

With a premed major in biology and a minor in chemistry, my goal remained to attend medical school after my undergraduate studies were complete—though I was equally committed to playing football. It wasn't always easy balancing a heavy academic workload and the added responsibilities of a student athlete. Between workouts and practice, the team obligations often occupied six hours per day. But despite that commitment, I maintained a 4.0 GPA. In fact, my father thought that my grades were so good that I should apply to medical school early.

Others were not so encouraging, including a philosophy professor who told me I would "never get into medical school early." In fact, throughout my academic life, there were many who told me that I was reaching for the unattainable. But I knew I wasn't.

I was thrilled when, in 1992 during my third year of undergraduate studies, I was accepted into the University of Texas Medical School in San Antonio. It was my first-choice medical school due to the proximity to my family. Considering that Texas State wasn't exactly known as an academic powerhouse, I couldn't believe I got into a medical school with no undergraduate degree, which was almost unheard of.*

I still had two years of eligibility for football, but with the guarantee of entering medical school, the decision to leave my undergraduate studies came easy. I immediately called my parents to notify them of the great news. My mother could not have been prouder. My father happily took credit for the great idea. Meanwhile, my philosophy professor was visibly embarrassed by the news in light of his previous prediction.

Thinking back, it's hard to swallow the notion that a teacher or mentor would actually become a detractor or even an obstacle to a student's advancement. I discovered that some teachers could

---

* Since I qualified for the combined BS MD program, I was granted my BS after my first year in medical school.

even become jealous and resentful if you accomplished more than they did at a comparable age. You might assume they would be proud that their pupil excelled. Surprisingly, this happened to me at multiple stages in my education.

In high school, I had a 3.96 GPA rather than a 4.0, only because I got a B- in typing, of all classes, for "talking too much"! Otherwise, I had all As and took all AP courses. In college, multiple people told me I would never get into medical school early, and my football coach assumed I was too academic to be a starting running back. In medical school, the nerdy doctors thought I was a muscle head—too athletic to be a successful medical student. Later, during my residency, two spine professors decided they didn't like me personally because my wife made more money than they did. They predicted that I would never get into a good spine fellowship program, despite my excellent performance and in-training examinations score. They were all wrong. I ignored their negative commentary and never stopped trying. I learned to not be constrained by others' lack of foresight or support.

When those people discouraged me or even actively blocked me, it forced me to trust in myself and to trust in God too. Through sheer will and God's grace, I proved them all wrong. I truly believe that God had a very clear hand in opening pathways for me that seemed closed off and blocked. I learned to use my failures as fuel for a harder push toward my goals. I found alternative pathways by continuing to be diligent and faithful and to never give in. There *is* a plan for us all. We don't always accomplish what we expect when we expect it, but I believe things will work out better than we imagined if we lean on God. However, it will happen in God's time, not ours.

Years later, I would tell my four kids to approach life the same way: Always believe in yourself. Work hard. Pay attention to the details. Have faith. And when you hit a wall, drive harder or go around, but don't ever collapse or give up. Eventually the wall will break, and you will break *through* it. Bottom line: A life with no limitations begins in your own head, not in the opinions of others. So give no credence to those who minimize you. We were all created for greatness. You just have to believe that and unlock your potential.

A lesson for anyone who has ever been discouraged by the limited thinking and capabilities of others: Never allow anyone to write your story or determine the narrative of your life. Never let someone else's opinion of you dictate your opinion of yourself or your future success. Never allow anyone's personal flaws to become an obstacle to *your* success. They may be projecting onto you their own sense of personal failure.

Maybe my experience as a running back helped me form this early determination to defy the odds. Anytime I got discouraged by another person's negative opinion of me, I could always visualize putting my head down, hitting the wall, driving through the line, and never giving up until I broke into the open field toward the end zone. By putting myself in that frame of mind, I could access the inner drive and perseverance I needed to prove my naysayers wrong. I could excel despite them. This is the dogged determination that enabled me to face my enemies and opposition and to continue pushing forward toward my end goal of proving them wrong. Challenges and turmoil require strength and determination. Like my father, I don't back down from a challenge. I will not let someone's willpower overcome my own. You cannot let the detractors win.

Later, during my challenges as a physician, this mindset ensured my success. I had more to lose than my opponents did. I had more to gain from proving my innocence, and I was not willing to let them destroy me with money-driven lies. One of the keys to success is to keep getting up when you fall down. Eventually your opponent will give up or give in.

Right around the time I started college, my father began practicing as a counseling psychologist. In admiration of his accomplishment, I initially thought that I would become a psychiatrist so that we could open up a father–son practice. But in my first year of college, a torn ACL (anterior cruciate ligament) in my knee forced me to undergo reconstructive surgery—a potentially career-ending injury for a running back. This experience led to a sudden change of plans.

In the course of my surgery and rehabilitation, I was amazed by what the orthopaedic surgeon was able to do. With incredible precision, he had turned my knee "bionic." After just six months, I recovered completely and went right back to being a running back, just as good as ever—able to run *fast*, take a hit, and play.

I was so impressed by what the orthopaedic surgeon had done for my knee that I immediately decided I was going to become an orthopaedic surgeon. I thought to myself, *This is the kind of medicine I want to practice—something where I can intervene and definitively* fix *something.*

Once I was accepted into medical school and determined my specialty of choice, I had to start thinking about how I'd pay for it all. Medical students usually take out massive loans in the neighborhood of $350,000 or more by the time we graduate from medical school. Instead of accruing that kind of burdensome debt, my father suggested that applying for a U.S. Air Force Health

Professions Scholarship would be the perfect solution. I would get a sterling education, provide service to my country, and never pay for any of it. But as I found out, getting that military scholarship was a competitive process—and I *would* end up paying for my education, albeit in a different way.

In fact, the commitment to the U.S. Air Force in "exchange" for tuition was a bit of a trick, and it was rather deceiving for a naïve medical student. While they tell you it's a four-year commitment for a four-year scholarship, it doesn't really work that way. The clock on repayment (with your freedom, not your checkbook) begins once you're on active-duty service *after* residency training. What they don't tell you is that you have to do your training *first*, then you pay back the cost of those first four years as a staff doctor later. Also, every step of specialized training that you add on pushes the commitment time even further ahead. That's how my time commitment extended from four years of active duty service to fourteen before I was even eligible to separate from the military!

In any case, the Air Force was very particular about the students who were given a scholarship. Few scholarships were granted, so academic standards were quite high. Applicants had to obtain letters of recommendation from high-ranking military officers, U.S. senators, and college professors. We also had to write lengthy essays and undergo extensive in-person interviews.

But in 1992, I was awarded a U.S. Air Force Health Professions Scholarship, entering the inactive reserves as a second lieutenant medical student. As the routine developed, every summer between years in medical school, I would serve active duty, rotating through different departments and undergoing training in preparation for active-duty service. For all of my rotations, I chose Wilford

Hall—our flagship hospital and the biggest Air Force hospital in the country. Fortunately, my medical school and Wilford Hall were both in San Antonio, adding significant convenience to my summer rotations.

I'd compare my experience learning in medical school to drinking water from a fire hydrant. The sheer volume of information we were expected to absorb, memorize, and regurgitate was almost unfathomable and could nearly "drown" you. To this day, I look back at the way we were taught and am glad that most medical school programs have transitioned away from the two years of classroom learning with no clinical exposure. The new curriculum introduces medical students to the clinical environment early on. I think this is a good move, but I still believe there is too little emphasis on running a successful practice and the business of medicine.

Instead of obsessing over multiple-choice quizzes, as it does, medical school should focus on the ability to think critically and compassionately. You need to memorize all the facts, but you also need to think about patients as individuals, rather than them being just textbook cases. That's why being forced to answer those endless multiple-choice questions was ridiculous. We weren't performing seals. Such "testmanship" and the ability to academically grandstand is an inadequate way to discern a student's true knowledge, which is much better determined by essay-answered questions in my opinion.

Yet, I think most doctors become so focused on the textbook explanations that they are unable to *apply* that abstract knowledge to actual patients, whose diagnoses are as variable as people themselves. As I quickly found out during clinical rotations, every patient responds quite differently to interventions, medications, and treatments. Textbooks are a guideline, not a concrete source of accurate information for every diagnosis nor patient.

In short, beyond the clinical knowledge, which must become secondhand, it's an art to take those facts and creatively think outside the box. You need to identify complex diagnoses and formulate the proper medical or surgical interventions.

To face the demands of the material, as I quickly found out, almost everyone studied four hours a day during the week and eight hours a day on weekends. The intensity of it was humbling and eye-opening, to say the least. Everyone around me was top of their class and highly driven. Some were sincere and genuine and would become lifelong friends and allies, whereas others were willing to sabotage their classmates to get ahead.

Out of 125 students in my class, I had two close friends. One of them was Kwabena Owusu from Ghana; he had entered medical school at the advanced age of thirty-eight. We called him Kay. He had a raspy voice with an African accent. And although I'm not sure he was always trying to be funny, he was quite hilarious. Everything he said just came out with a unique twist to it. Crass as he was, fortunately (for him), he was married to an elegant British–Ghanian woman, Sylvia, who was as lovely as her accent.

But my closest friend was Joseph Puente, a graduate of Baylor College who was very well prepared and adept in the classroom. Joey, as we called him, was a whiz. His ability to answer multiple-choice questions correctly was impressive. When we were studying together, I often didn't feel that his answers made sense. But Joey had great natural instincts and would say, "I could be wrong, but what I said just feels like the right answer." When we started our clinical rotations, I was convinced that our preceptors would always give Joey a slightly higher mark than me because he looked like the stereotypical medical student (thin with glasses), whereas I looked like a jock—a bulky 235 pounds.

Together, the three of us—Kay, Joey, and I—became quite close and studied often together, quizzing each other before phase exams. Trust me, I needed as much quizzing as possible. Having only attended three years of college, it was obvious that I was at a definite disadvantage. Many of my classmates already had their master's or doctorate degrees, and all of them had their bachelor's degrees. Some of them were nurses or therapists, or even doctors, who were clearly familiar with the material; whereas I was a guy with three years of undergraduate experience, looking at massive volumes of information for the very first time.

One of my most inspirational (and entertaining) professors was the dean of students, Carlos Pestana—an elegant Spaniard who was a general surgeon and a very engaging lecturer. Through him, I better understood the complexities of the patient–doctor relationship and the subtleties of treatments to be considered.

As the workload and training unfolded, my second year of medical school was almost the death of me, literally. One day, I came down with the most severe headache of my life. It felt as if a bomb was going off in the back of my head. In addition, I had a 103-degree fever and an incredibly stiff neck. Worst of all, I was vomiting about fifty times a day. I went to the emergency department on three different occasions and explained to the doctors that I believed I had meningitis.

Unfortunately, the fact that I was a medical student actually worked against me. The running joke is that when all of us learn about each disease, we start developing those very symptoms. It's actually kind of true. But in this case, I had become delirious from the electrolyte imbalance after a week of nonstop vomiting and continued fever. Yet the Stanford-trained ER doctor erroneously dismissed my claims and sent me home with a diagnosis of *cephalgia* (a fancy way to say headache).

Thankfully, a new ER doctor ultimately performed the correct evaluation and determined that I did have symptoms consistent with meningitis and that I needed a lumbar puncture, which is when a needle is inserted into the spinal nerve sac to aspirate spinal fluid. Once I was accurately diagnosed with meningitis, I was admitted immediately to an isolation room and given IV antibiotics. The initial incompetence of my diagnosis was a great lesson, demonstrating that doctors are no less subject to human error than anyone else—even those trained at illustrious institutions! This experience also taught me to *listen* to my patients. Even the best doctors make mistakes and miss diagnoses. It's important to hear what your patients tell you and to investigate their assumptions, even if they seem unlikely. Even with my experience and background, there have been many instances in which a patient told me something about their condition that seemed far-fetched, but I listened to their concerns. I discovered several issues that I nor anyone else would have likely caught based on medical probabilities, had I ignored my patient.

By the time I recovered enough to return to medical school, I had missed six weeks of classes. By this point, final examinations were coming up and—though I tried hard to function well—I struggled to read and concentrate. I still had the pounding headaches, plus I now had blurry vision too. I spoke with my professors about it and was informed that if I was unable to take the final examinations, I would be forced to repeat the year.

I refused to consider that option and buried my head in the books all hours of the day and night, barreling through and attempting to cram six weeks of information into my pounding, foggy brain. Though I inwardly conceded that I might fail for the first time in my life...I didn't. My hard work paid off. I didn't get an A in every class, but I passed and avoided the dread of repeating another year. I realized that all As didn't necessarily define a successful student. Many doctors with stellar grades fail to translate their testing skills into real-world application. I have seen many doctors who finished at the top of their classes but were subpar clinicians or surgeons. I realized that things happen outside of your control sometimes. True success comes from the ability to pick yourself up from failures or setbacks and to drive forward. Setbacks create strength and build willpower. In the end, success is even sweeter when the path was more difficult along the way.

However, the negative impact of meningitis on my overall GPA presented a whole new challenge. After all, I still planned to apply for an orthopaedic residency, which is one of the most competitive of them all. And getting in with a chink in my academic armor would not be so easy.

As I entered the third year of medical school—now interacting with patients in clinic and hospital settings—I felt a sense of increased confidence. Up until then, I had found our classroom regimen unnecessarily laborious, but assimilating what I had learned came pretty easily to me. During these clinical rotations, I really began to excel. I was fortunate to have a number of brilliant surgical specialists who were training me, though not always with a subtle touch.

At the time, the department of orthopaedics at the University of Texas Health Science Center at San Antonio was ranked number five in the country. There was a famous shoulder surgeon there named Charlie Rockwood. He was a character. He was known for his casual southern demeanor, quick wit, and comedic talents just as much as his surgical skills. He and a hand surgeon named David Green authored what was considered the "bible of orthopaedic surgery"—*Rockwood and Green's Fractures in Adults*. This duo had a lot to do with the stellar reputation of the program.

Dr. Rockwood's protégé and partner was a shoulder surgeon named Michael Wirth. He was nicknamed the "velvet hammer." Though he was soft-spoken, his searing criticisms of the residents would nonetheless destroy their egos. He had the most melodic and soothing voice imaginable, but his feedback was laced with disdain. However, despite his sometimes harsh critiques, he was a superb surgeon who never mistreated me. In fact, I learned an immense amount from both Dr. Rockwood and Dr. Wirth. They both had a great bedside manner and always treated patients with humility and care.

It was not all pleasant, however. The total joint surgeon at the time, who shall remain nameless, had an enormous head—literally and figuratively. He was my first encounter with what we refer to in medicine as a "malignant personality." This describes a staff physician who is unnecessarily condescending and disrespectful of students and residents. My first, and thankfully last, experience with him was when he yelled at me for crossing my arms after scrubbing in for surgery. As a surgeon now, I know he was wrong. I hadn't contaminated myself, but I was terrified at the time that I had done something gravely wrong and was compromising the sterility of the operating room.

Thankfully, counterbalancing that experience was Dr. Fred Corley, who was one of the gems of the department. He was a burly southern gentleman—a former Ole Miss lineman who was one of the nicest staff surgeons I've ever met. He was also hardworking beyond anything you could imagine. We would catch him at three in the morning mopping up the floor because someone had spilled a drink on the stairs leading from the operating room to the ER!

We always chuckled when he would confer with us after patient rounds. In his thick southern drawl, he'd ask, "Did you tell them they could die?" Although it was extreme for most patients we saw, he was right to lay out all the possibilities. So often physicians sugarcoated the possible outcomes of surgery, which was something he never did, nor do I. If a patient has unreasonable expectations, it can create major problems.

I loved my rotations, especially the ones in the orthopaedic department. While on call at nights, there was an air of excitement—a looming expectation that we would be able to help multiple injured patients who walked through our doors. One of my favorite experiences was reducing (realigning) dislocated joints and fractures or stabilizing broken or dislocated bones. I never seemed to get tired of doing it, even though I was existing on almost no sleep at the time.

One thing we never learned, despite four years of condensed learning on any and everything that ails the body and mind, was business. We didn't have a single course or even lecture about the subject of business. Thus, we graduated with zero business acumen. Our first two years of lectures were focused on anatomy, physiology, microbiology, pharmacology, neurosciences, pathology, etc., but nothing related to private practice. In hindsight, that's an enormous mistake that has made all physicians vulnerable to innumerable business disasters.

At the time I graduated from medical school in 1996, I applied for acceptance into several orthopaedic residency programs nationwide, all of which were highly competitive. As I discovered, the military has rigid quotas about how many surgeons they will allow to seek this specialty training. At the time I applied, the chairman of the Air Force orthopaedic department, Ken Kaylor, had miscalculated the correct number of slots available, denying the ability of thirty-two medical students to apply for a civilian orthopaedic residency—including me! Unfortunately, this mistake was made after we had all spent time and money traveling to interviews to find the perfect civilian training program.

In my disappointment, I turned to my father, who recommended I write asking for a congressional inquiry about the Air Force's decision. I penned letters to two Texas senators and one representative, in addition to President Bill Clinton himself. It turned out that my plea fell mostly on deaf ears. Only our local congressman, Frank Tejeda—a former Marine—lifted a finger to help, but he was unsuccessful. None of the others even bothered to respond.

You might be wondering why I was so upset by Kaylor's decision to block us from accepting a civilian orthopaedic residency. For starters, we had been told that 90 percent of doctors were given their first choice of residency training. I had busted my hump in medical school with the goal of fulfilling my dream, one that was now being derailed. In my mind, I was on the fast track, having graduated med school in only three years, but now my train was off the track. By denying our ability to enter a civilian orthopaedic program out of medical school, it would mean a minimum of two additional years spent in the field waiting for a new position to open up (either in a civilian program or the only military program at Wilford Hall). Even more frustrating was that the students who graduated the year following us were able to apply for orthopaedic surgery programs unimpeded by any restrictive entrance quotas, making that year even more competitive than usual. In fact, there were thirty-six open positions for the graduating class the year behind us; and many of them went unfilled!

During the time I was awaiting the Air Force's determination on the number of slots that would be permitted, I had been offered a position in the orthopaedic residency at Albert Einstein Montefiore in New York. I was still awaiting the decision of the other programs. While I had hoped the pressure of my congressional inquiry would allow me to accept the orthopaedic residency that I had been offered, the Air Force had other plans. I received a no-nonsense letter from the general who was the head of assignments at Randolph Air Force Base, ordering the following: "Lieutenant Cyr must and will report to Wilford Hall as directed." That statement sealed my fate. I would not be allowed to pursue civilian training. As a military asset, your ability to enter civilian training versus military training, or the specialty of your choice, is at the sole discretion of the military. If the powers that be decide that you cannot train in a civilian program, even if they had allowed it for ten years prior, you will not train in a civilian program. You go where they say, when they say. I realized I may have created a future backlash for my persistence. I also came to understand I was no longer free to do as I pleased. I was no longer free at all.

This meant that I would now be going into a one-year transitional/rotating internship at Wilford Hall. I had preemptively applied for that position once I realized the opportunity for orthopaedics may not come to fruition. I always had a backup plan. Yes, it was a great internship, but it was unaffiliated with an orthopaedic residency, which was my dream. It was a rotating internship in which the interns rotated through different specialties to gain an understanding of multiple fields. This meant that once the internship was complete, I would have to either apply for an orthopaedic residency position in a civilian program again (repeating the internship year) or get into a second-year spot, of which there were very few in the country—including the one at Wilford Hall, which was ultra-competitive. At this point, my best option was the Air Force's sole orthopaedic surgery program at Wilford Hall, which only accepted four residents per year. That was obviously my new goal, and I had to grease the wheels big-time to get into it.

So, as a super-busy intern who was rotating through every department of the hospital, I also acted as a gopher, volunteering to carry the call pagers for the orthopaedic residents. I also offered to perform their scut work, such as getting lab results, checking on patients, and changing dressings.

One thing the internship at Wilford Hall did was position me to be in the hospital where the military program was housed. So, despite the impossibly heavy workload, one major benefit of the transitional year was that it gave me additional elective rotations, which I used to spend more time in the orthopaedic surgery department. It also allowed me to meet and get to know the orthopaedic residents and staff and to attend their morning conferences, but all my efforts to get into the Air Force orthopaedic residency would be a steep challenge. Little did I know that it was the orthopaedic chairman *at Wilford Hall*, Colonel Kaylor, who was forced to answer the congressional inquiries I had generated in my attempt to get authorization to attend a civilian orthopaedic residency. This was obviously extra work for and an embarrassment to him, making me his *least* favorite candidate for consideration into the program.

Luckily, while in medical school, I began performing

orthopaedic research at Wilford Hall for Dr. Michael Yaszemski, a Harvard-trained spinal surgeon who was quite an imposing guy, formerly an offensive tackle at Lehigh University. Thankfully, he took a liking to me and became a strong advocate for my application to the Air Force's orthopaedic residency.

Unfortunately, Dr. Yaszemski and Dr. Kaylor did not get along at all. In fact, the chairman had a history of attempting to block any of Dr. Yaszemski's protégés from acceptance into the Air Force's orthopaedic residency.

Not surprisingly, Kaylor had already openly stated that I would never get into his Air Force orthopaedic residency program, but somehow God literally moved him out of the way, as he was involuntarily separated from the military immediately prior to my application. I never heard the explanation of *how* this had happened, but, trust me, it is extremely uncommon for any medical officer to be removed from active service.

With Dr. Kaylor out of the way, I was accepted into the orthopaedic residency program in 1997 for a position beginning in 1999.

After my internship, while I awaited my residency slot, I attended aerospace medicine training and became a flight surgeon assigned to Lackland Air Force Base, adjacent to Wilford Hall. This proximity allowed me to continue attending orthopaedic morning conferences while also carrying the call pagers. As I see it now, this two-year hiatus became an enormous blessing for me because it allowed me the freedom in my schedule to meet LeAnn (again). I can't tell you how many times I prayed that I could get in to a civilian program out of medical school. It didn't happen, but God had a different plan. It's funny how life works out.

Often our immediate desires are not met because God has a grander plan in mind for us, something bigger and better than we could even imagine for ourselves. It's these delays in gratification—the challenges we face along the way, the failures, trials, and turmoil—that bring true joy to our victories in the end. We may not accomplish what we originally set out to accomplish, but I believe God is steering us to a more glorious result if we keep the faith.

Chapter Five

A Cinderella Story

It was during my two years as a flight surgeon at Lackland Air Force Base from 1997 to 1999 that I was reintroduced to LeAnn, the girl from the Philippines who I had not seen in fourteen years. Since my senior year of college, I had been in a committed relationship—though it was a tumultuous one. We just weren't right for each other and argued frequently. After seven years, I finally realized I was wasting both our time, so we finally went our separate ways.

Right around that time, my older brother Bryan attended a reunion in Las Vegas for alumni from our old high school on Clark Air Base in the Philippines. After it ended, for whatever reason, Bryan left my contact information behind as a way for attendees to contact him. One day, my brother's ex-girlfriend from the Philippines, Maria, called me looking for him. I connected her to Bryan, and they reminisced about how LeAnn had a crush on me and how perfect we would be together.

Fortuitously, Maria had remained close friends with LeAnn. So after some deliberation, my brother and Maria decided to play matchmaker. Bryan insisted I call LeAnn. I was typically shy, but one day I just took a chance and called her. Prior to that call, I had never approached a girl without knowing beforehand that she was already interested in me. But I figured I really had nothing to lose, as I had already spent seven years with the wrong person.

At that time, LeAnn was living in Fort Lauderdale and had been thriving as a corporate recruiter. Impressively, at the age of only twenty-six, she was working for a Fortune 1000 company and already bringing in a six-figure income. She had been loving life in south Florida with a great group of other professional, single women. They were all successful and young and unattached. She lived in the art deco district of Fort Lauderdale on Las Olas Boulevard, surrounded by Cuban restaurants, nonstop music, and positive vibes. She was a simple person with few lofty expectations. She lived in an efficiency apartment within walking distance to many of her favorite hotspots and the beach!

When I first called her, it was slightly awkward. After all, it had been fourteen years.

"Do you remember me?" I asked with some irony. Her response was, "Yeah, I remember you. You were mean and said I had stinky feet and a deep voice. I'm still going through counseling because of what you said to me!"

I loved that she had a sense of humor. Though I knew she was joking with me, I still felt terrible and immediately apologized. What ensued after that icebreaker was the most amazing two-hour conversation. We talked about her childhood, our families, our mutual experiences in the Philippines, and the friends we had in common. And then, as a lot of children of foreign mothers do, we impersonated our mothers and laughed about it!

It was obvious that there was an instant emotional connection, and I felt a sense of commonality that I had never felt before. LeAnn was intelligent and witty, totally engaging and very funny. She had a very distinctive DC inflection, almost as if I was speaking to Thurston Howell's daughter. She was obviously highly intelligent but also self-effacing. As I learned, she had attended George Mason University and completed her graduate assistantship studies at Georgetown.

The conversation that night was so amazing that I was very reluctant to end it, and I didn't take very long to call her up again. Let's just say that I was never very good at poker.

The next time we connected over the phone, we had another engaging conversation. She knew how interested I was, and I was doing nothing to hide it. I was not the type to play games and didn't plan on being anything but honest with her. Later I would find out that she found this to be incredibly refreshing.

Almost every night for the next month we talked over the phone; each conversation lasted two hours at a minimum. I was totally infatuated. All day long, I would think about my upcoming call that night and couldn't wait to hear her voice again. In truth, I had already fallen in love with her over the phone.

I asked her every question I wanted to know about a prospective life partner. We discussed our faith, the number of children we thought would be ideal, who would handle the finances in a marriage, whether we believed in prenuptial agreements, if we would want joint checking accounts, etc.

We talked about working mothers versus stay-at-home mothers. I explained to her that I would support whatever she wanted to do. I truly believe motherhood is the most important responsibility on the planet. I told her that if she chose to stay home with kids, I would work three jobs to support our family, but also if she wanted to continue working, I would support that as well.

At this time, of course, she was making way more money than I was—even though I had been moonlighting downtown at three different primary care clinics. No matter what we talked about, she checked every box! I was totally in love and convinced that she was the woman for me. Whether it was accident or fate, God's will or luck, we had to now meet in person!

So we decided to create a mini-reunion, a one-week trip to Fort Lauderdale that would include Maria and my brother and LeAnn and me.

I still remember that plane ride so vividly, sitting next to my brother and looking out the window trying to imagine what LeAnn looked like after *fourteen* years. The last time I had seen her at age twelve, she was rail thin and taller than me. Her hair was lightened with peroxide—a typical eighties look. When I conjured up a picture of her, I could still see her soft smile and kind eyes. All in all, she was really an adorable Amerasian girl who was quite shy.

Maria bragged to my brother about how LeAnn had blossomed into a "bombshell with brains." I was excited to see her! Prior to the trip, LeAnn had asked me to describe *myself*. And so I did, telling her that I went from being a short five-foot, 100-pound thirteen-year-old to five foot eleven and 225 pounds, having bulked up from weightlifting and football over the years. Yet all she could remember was the much shorter version of me with chubby cheeks and my hair slicked back, always sweating from breaking and popping.

It felt like a blind date was about to happen, so it was nerve-wracking. After all, people change a lot in fourteen years. This was before the era of social media, when we could have had a Zoom call or easily scoped out photos of each other.

Yet we intentionally decided *not* to exchange pictures. What we had between us by phone was so pure and real that we did not want to undermine it with superficiality. It was definitely a risk. But like I said, I had already fallen in love with who LeAnn was on the phone. So, if we had any physical chemistry at all, I was already confident I would want to *marry* her. Although I was only twenty-seven at the time, I definitely felt ready to start married life with the right person. I already could tell she was my soulmate.

Upon landing, as we walked through the airport—and even from a distance—I recognized LeAnn immediately. She was wearing a form-fitting copper-colored dress and was *visually amazing*. In a split second when I saw her, I knew deep in my heart that I was going to marry her. After a very short period of awkwardness, things fell right into place. We began talking and joking around just as if we had last seen each other a few weeks earlier. It was as if time had stopped, and we just picked up where we left off.

By our third day together, I was madly in love with LeAnn. Based upon the look on her face, I think the feeling was mutual. Up until this point, as I learned, LeAnn had been in a number of failed relationships, which were no different than mine. There was much frustration and disappointment on both sides.

As she remembers it, "At twenty-six years old, I was not holding my breath for a sincere, handsome, successful, and intelligent person to come around. I had pretty much resigned myself that being alone is better than being in bad company. In fact, I think my parents thought I would grow old alone and would wind up to be an old maid. But from my perspective, it was hard to find someone who could handle my strong personality. I'm an alpha female and can be very set in my ways and driven, especially back then.

"But Steven's personality was the perfect complement to mine, because he is extremely passive—in a good way. He doesn't let little things bother him, and he certainly is not going to argue with me about mundane things. He has more important things to worry about, like people's lives!"

As for me, I knew for sure that we were perfect from the start, and we were soon talking about marriage. By the time I had to return to San Antonio, we both shed tears at the thought of being apart, even though we had only been reunited for a month. The phone calls continued nonstop, and by December, LeAnn invited me to her family's home in northern Virginia to meet her parents.

LeAnn's mother, Carol, was the life of the party—bubbly and energetic and so welcoming. Her characteristic Vietnamese accent was intermittently accentuated by uproarious laughter and constant joking. She kept saying what I thought was, "I'm Ron Riva!" Eventually, I realized she was saying Joan Rivers. She was hilarious and sweet. The day I arrived, she actually came to the airport to pick me up with a cooler full of Vietnamese spring rolls and other snacks and drinks. Her father, Jack, was an imposing man who stood at six foot four; he was quiet and quite serious—the exact opposite of his wife. It didn't take long for Carol to take me aside and confide that LeAnn had come very close to marrying a cardiologist, and that it was a good thing that I came along when I did. Later I would find out that this was a total exaggeration to make me aware of how special her daughter was. I didn't need any convincing. I was in it for life.

During that trip, I fell in love with my future in-laws too. LeAnn's father jokingly told me that she was so picky that he thought she would wind up being an old maid. He confided that he was incredibly happy that I came along.

On this trip, out of respect, I asked LeAnn's father for his permission to have her hand in marriage, even though we had only been dating for three months. He granted it. Right after that, Carol and I drove to a Vietnamese jewelry shop, where we picked out a beautiful three-carat marquise stone. Thanks to Carol's friendship with the owner, I was given the rock-bottom price of $8,000.

Considering what I was getting, it was a great deal—though it would take months for me to pay for it, which I did by increasing my moonlighting hours. One of the clinics I worked at was an urgent care clinic located right next to a nightclub with music that blasted throughout the night. On weekends, it was bit torturous hearing the constant thump of the beat as I tried to gain a couple of hours of sleep prior to my next shift. But as I constantly reminded myself, I was doing it for an extremely important cause.

To provide myself a bit of comfort, I would call LeAnn's work phone in the middle of the night just so that I could hear her voice on her answering machine. That alone would give me continued motivation.

I also worked at both an urgent care center, WellMed, in a quieter part of town, and at Gamboa Family Practice. Dr. Jose Gamboa was a dignified man and an extremely busy physician who was well-liked by everyone. I really enjoyed working for him.

By April 1999, I had earned enough money to pay for the ring. That month, LeAnn was being awarded with a "top earners" trip to Disney World, a gift from her company for being in the top 5 percent among her fellow headhunters, and she invited me as her guest on the trip.

On the plane ride to Orlando, I just happened to sit next to a Disney employee. When I shared with him my intention to ask LeAnn to marry me, he helped me create the perfect proposal plan, suggesting that I propose at the wedding pavilion overlooking the lake near Cinderella's Castle.

When we got to the Disney gift shop, I immediately bought a small crystal Cinderella slipper and had it engraved with the date: *April 9, 1999, Steven & LeAnn*. I lined the inside of the slipper with black felt and then placed the ring inside it. Then I got a large box to disguise it, because I knew the weight of the container would throw LeAnn off and confuse her even more. I wanted it to be a complete surprise.

On April 9, 1999, after dinner at the Grand Floridian, we headed toward the wedding pavilion, where I noticed three kids waiting on the steps to see the fireworks over Cinderella's Castle. I bent over and told them that I was going to ask LeAnn to marry me. The kids were so sweet; without saying anything further, they quietly left us alone. At nine o'clock when the fireworks began, I bent down on one knee and I proposed, telling LeAnn that all my life I had been looking for *my* Cinderella. "I'm now sure that I have finally found her... I know the slipper is a perfect fit."

She said yes! As she remembers it now, "I was surprised by how sweet and sentimental he was, though I shouldn't have been, because he was like that throughout our courtship."

Needless to say, we were both elated, sharing fireworks of our own as we embarked on a brand-new life together.

Just a month after the trip to Disneyland, LeAnn moved from Florida to Texas to start planning the December 18 wedding. That summer, I was beginning my much-awaited residency, making 1999 a pivotal year in many ways.

After conferring with her mother at length, LeAnn decided to travel to Vietnam to purchase her wedding gown (made by a local seamstress in her mother's hometown for $200!) and everything else we needed—including the bridesmaids' gowns, groomsmen's tuxedos, and invitations. We got it all at a fraction of the cost they would have been in the States. In the end, while the wedding seemed quite extravagant, it was surprisingly inexpensive.

On the day of our wedding, as LeAnn and I entered the Incarnate Word Motherhouse Chapel in San Antonio, we were both awestruck. It was all pale marble with gold accents and stained-glass-filtered light. I felt happier than I had ever been.

As LeAnn recalls, "Steve, who is ordinarily so calm and composed in the OR, was the more emotional one at the wedding. One of my mom's friends said that she had never seen a man cry so much in her entire life. In fact, this has become an ongoing joke in our family, embellished to make Steve look as over-sensitive as possible!"

After the service, the wedding reception was held at a venue that overlooked the city and the riverwalk, and we arranged river boat barge rides for all our guests. At the end of the night, LeAnn and I rode off in a horse-drawn Cinderella carriage—followed by a quick honeymoon to Jamaica.

After the honeymoon, I returned to my residency. LeAnn continued to work in corporate recruiting. She switched companies after moving from Fort Lauderdale to San Antonio. She earned even more at the new company, making us very comfortable financially, even though I was a resident.

Even with this added comfort, there were a few bumps at the start of our marriage. As LeAnn remembers it, "Some of the problems in the beginning of our marriage revolved around my future in-laws and I coming to an understanding that our marriage was between the two of us and not between us and all of them. Steve came from a very close family, as did I. But the difference between them was that my family is very careful not to cross social boundaries with each other; whereas with Steve's family, there were few boundaries.

"So, this took a little bit of adjustment for me and them. I wasn't used to being told what to do, how to live my life, and how to handle my finances at twenty-six years old. After all, I had been doing just fine on my own up until then. I was very successful and independent. I had been earning a salary well into the six figures since finishing grad school. I felt like I didn't need a lot of financial advice."

There was no doubt in my mind that LeAnn could certainly take care of herself! Her strength and independence would later benefit our marriage immensely. My career would require many late nights and many missed engagements/events. LeAnn had to be comfortable without my making it to dinner many nights. Oftentimes, this is a source of great distress in the lives of physicians and their spouses. A successful marriage requires the spouse to be independent enough to understand the weight of the job that keeps their husband or wife at work at the expense of family time. Her strength was also imperative if we were to confront the legal and professional battles we were about to face. I can only imagine how different the result would have been if I wasn't married to a strong and intelligent woman.

Chapter Six

Surgical Precision

In July of 1999, I began my orthopaedic residency. I can't even begin to explain how excited I was to marry the woman of my dreams and for my dreams of becoming an orthopaedic surgeon to be coming to fruition. On the hospital front, my orthopaedic residency was turning out to be an intriguing experience, to say the least. The new chairman of the department, Ted Parsons, was a Harvard-trained musculoskeletal oncologist—probably the most complicated subspecialty within orthopaedics. He was a brilliant surgeon and quite an imposing man, at six foot seven, as tall as he was talented. As I learned, he was also a priest in the Church of Jesus Christ of Latter-Day Saints and highly devoted to his faith, which was evident in the way he treated others (including me, as he turned out to be a phenomenal mentor).

His focus on academics for our residency ensured it would be one of the top-rated programs in the country. In fact, under his guidance, residents would consistently score in the top 5 percent in the nation on their in-training examinations. Dr. Parsons was an academic giant, embodying everything an orthopaedic surgeon should aspire to be. He was conscientious, humble, strict, driven, attentive to details, meticulous, and brilliant.

Even under the best of circumstances, residency is not without its physical and emotional challenges. During our trauma rotation, which we performed at the University of Texas Health Science Center, we were expected to work on call every other night. Demanding 120-hour workweeks continued for months at a time. This meant that we would be up for *forty* hours at a time, followed by four hours of sleep before the next shift. Meanwhile, well-meaning nurses would call us up at all hours of the night with questions and requests. Although this was challenging, it forced us to learn how to work meticulously (although exhausted) and how to push ourselves beyond what we thought were our limits. Why did we do it? Because the reward of our job was visible and oftentimes almost immediate, and we really had no choice. This is the life of a surgeon.

The excitement of being on call for highly complicated cases was that we were able to fix broken bones that had punctured through the skin; reduce (realign or put back into place) broken bones and dislocated joints; and treat all types of injuries of the musculoskeletal system. Getting outstanding results was one of the most rewarding parts of the job; it definitely outweighed the burden of the administrative follow-up and lack of sleep.

After residency started, there was an interesting dynamic at Wilford Hall that began to brew. The staff surgeons were a mix of civilian-trained and military-trained orthopaedic specialists. The hierarchy in the military is extraordinarily strong. It created a perplexing medical culture in which nurses could outrank doctors.

Because the Air Force's interests came first and foremost, it was a little bit of a socialist environment in which everyone had to look the same, march the same, talk the same, and fit in. There were some very caustic personalities, which is commonplace in surgical specialties but can be even more compounded by military structure, rules, and regulations. I guess some people are so proud of themselves when they make it through medical school and the rigors of residency that they start to become a "little" egomaniacal.

Although what we do can be impressive and our responsibilities enormous, I never felt that way. When I got a pat on the back from a supervising surgeon or thanks from a grateful patient, I always felt as if *I* had been blessed—that God was the one who deserved the praise, not me.

It was during this intense period of training that my faith grew as I learned more about the intricate inner workings of the human body. I was awestruck and sometimes bewildered that trillions of cells could work synchronously to keep our bodies thriving. How in the world could this have been random chance? In other words, believing that God created man in his image, there was a definite spiritual component to my amazement and respect for the miracle of our bodies, and I felt privileged to be a physician.

However, many of my colleagues weren't so faith-focused. As in any large hospital setting, there are always competing factions of surgeons and residents, and some of their antics and personalities are quite off-putting. Some of the civilian-trained staff were actually the worst mentors (*and* people) I had ever met—they were totally full of themselves. Ironically, their surgical outcomes didn't justify their high opinions of themselves! They were also rather disrespectful to the military residents and even wore shirts off duty with the letters "IDARR." This stood for "I did a real residency." We certainly resented them for that, and if the residency was inferior, weren't they partly to blame? They were part of the teaching faculty.

Unfortunately, the quality of leadership began to deteriorate once Dr. Parsons left his role as chairman of orthopaedics in 2000, especially since Dr. Yaszemski had already left the Air Force prior to my even starting the residency in 1997 to take a staff position at the Mayo Clinic. As a result of their exits, the program dramatically declined, in my opinion, paving the way for less polished and academic chairmen to take Parsons's place. The impact of this bureaucratic change was only worsened by the devastating events of 9/11.

In the aftermath of 9/11, the hospital commander and surgeon general of the Air Force decided that the Air Force would become the "9-1-1 rescue squad to the world," a proactive expeditionary medical team. This would mean that Wilford Hall, the Air Force's flagship hospital (the final stop for battlefield injuries from overseas) would now turn into a mobile unit of medics and physicians traveling to the front lines of battle to provide more expedient care to servicemen and women injured in combat.

It was a grand plan that led the hospital commander to being selected as the next surgeon general, but ultimately it would ruin our residency program both academically and socially, creating a stressful environment for staff, who were always on edge about having to deploy to faraway spots on a moment's notice. Surgeons who were previously collegial began to turn on one another.

Any physician who had a medical diagnosis (like sleep apnea, asthma, or disc herniation, among many other conditions) would be ineligible for deployment. They became the pariahs of the department. Why? Because the unwanted deployments became even more frequent for other surgeons. Meanwhile, the staff surgeons were so busy deploying to Iraq and Afghanistan and then recovering from their assignments that little time was devoted to maintaining the high caliber of the teaching program.

In my fourth year of residency, I began preparing to apply to spine fellowship programs at many of the top hospitals in the country, but I was almost thwarted by two "malignant" staff spine surgeons (co-founders of the IDARR faction) who didn't like me personally. They had no reason to dislike me other than the fact that, at the time, my wife was earning more money than any of the staff surgeons in the hospital. Unfortunately, they found this out from a fellow resident who I had confided in after he repeatedly asked me how much money my wife was making. Bottom-line: these two surgeons decided that they would not support my application for the fellowship.

One of them, a Mayo-trained spine surgeon, actually had the audacity to flat-out tell me that (despite scoring in the top 4 percent in the nation) I would never get into the fellowship program at the Mayo Clinic. The fact that I was diligent and respectful made no difference.

Undaunted by this self-proclaimed clairvoyant, I was determined to prove both antagonists wrong. Like so many times before in my life, I refused to allow someone else to create a false narrative about me that would dash my dreams or obstruct my potential for success. I applied for a clinical rotation in the orthopaedic spine surgery department at the Mayo Clinic to prove my worth. I spent a month there working diligently to prove my skill and potential. My efforts paid off, and I *was* accepted.*

---

*   I was also offered a prestigious fellowship at the Weill Cornell Hospital for Special Surgery in New York. At the time, Mayo was rated number one, and—more importantly—it was a better fit for me.

In fact, I ended up being the *only* spine fellow at Mayo in their combined orthopaedic and neurosurgical spine fellowship, which would begin in the summer of 2003. To put me in an even better mood during that fall of 2001, LeAnn and I found out that she was pregnant. What a year! I had been accepted into the two top spine programs in the country, *and* we were having our first baby! I couldn't have been happier. From the time I was a kid, I had always dreamed of being a father. I loved babies and couldn't wait to raise my own with the woman I loved. This was truly the best time of my life.

The beautiful thing about the acceptance to Mayo was that it was timed perfectly, putting me in position to return to Wilford Hall as chief of spine surgery for the entire Air Force—a position that carried with it the title of consultant to the Air Force surgeon general and Pentagon.

My education at the Mayo Clinic was unparalleled. First of all, every person affiliated with Mayo beamed with pride to be part of such an amazing place. From the people mopping the floors to the heads of each department, the atmosphere was one of warmth and humility. The level of talent and brilliance of the staff—in addition to the sheer size of the main building—was awe-inspiring; I was trained by world-famous neurosurgeons and orthopaedists (though they casually introduced themselves by first name only), many of whom had developed their own implant systems. (In fact, their innovation and ingenuity foreshadowed creations of my own in years to come; more on that later.) In addition to their surgery and teaching, these physicians published numerous scientific papers while still making time to chair various spine organizations. One of the things I recognized that was different from most surgical departments was their methodical approach to patient evaluations. Despite the high demand for consultations, the volume of patients seen was kept to a reasonable number to allow for a thorough evaluation and attention to detail. This was no mill, and the conscientiousness of the physicians and staff was apparent.

As the only spine fellow, I took spine call every third night and performed complex multilevel spinal surgeries and reconstructions of all areas of the spine, from the base of the skull to the tailbone. I also presented at the weekly grand rounds, where I was quizzed by neurosurgery and orthopaedic spine specialists. They grilled me on my cases, quizzing me on journal articles, physical anatomy, and treatment options for each patient. It was the perfect balance between clinical training/teaching and operative experience and guidance. Many fellowships focus only on attaining surgical skills with little time devoted to the clinic setting. However, it's in the clinic where physicians learn to talk to, relate to, and to work up their patients' problems. Without adequate training in the clinical setting a surgeon may be very talented technically, but they are disastrous when it comes to interpersonal skills and the knowledge necessary to identify the source of a patient's problem. I believe that is why many surgeons who are extremely bright and skilled surgically have poor surgical outcomes. They don't know what surgery to perform to adequately eliminate or alleviate the problem. The ability to diagnose a problem through the correct workup of tests and examination findings comes from the knowledge attained in the clinic.

To be honest, I hadn't received very good training in spine surgery in my residency. I felt the Mayo Clinic and the Thomas

Jefferson–trained spine surgeons in my residency, who were very impressed with themselves, did a poor job of teaching spine surgery principles and techniques to the residents. Thus, I wasn't the strongest fellow starting out.

However, I devoted myself to learning all the specifics of spine surgery by preparing for clinic, surgery, lectures, weekly case conferences, and independent study beyond what was being demanded. In the end, with the guidance provided and my grit, I finished as a pretty capable spine surgeon. (Experts say it takes three to five years after fellowship to get a level of comfort and skill to develop true confidence in spine surgery; this is when one is forced to put their training to the test without someone guiding their every move.)

Most important was my observation of their world-class surgical skill, amplified by the use of cutting-edge technology and techniques. As I witnessed it in the OR, their surgical knowledge was unmatched by anything I had previously seen. To top it all off, these surgeons were even humble and gracious. This was quite different from those two obstructive bozos who had attempted to keep me from this opportunity. I grew exponentially as a surgeon and became very comfortable with the treatment of complex issues affecting the spine.

From a personal standpoint, I must say that Rochester, Minnesota, was both the coldest and warmest place I'd ever lived in. It was literally freezing in the winter, dropping down to -36 degrees. (We parked in an enclosed garage then entered the various buildings via subterranean pedestrian walkways to avoid freezing to death!) But the people in the hospital gave me the warmest welcome I'd ever received. Every single person I met was cheerful and enthusiastic, seemingly proud to be a part of this world-class institution. From the janitors to the chairmen of departments, everyone was gracious and kind.

On the home front, the winter of 2002 was quite challenging for LeAnn, who had always been accustomed to the warm temperatures of Florida and Texas. To her, Minnesota felt like Antarctica. However, when summer finally dawned, just before I had begun my fellowship, our newborn daughter, Alexa, arrived. She was such a startlingly beautiful baby; she had piercing blue eyes that you could see from across the room. Everywhere we went, women would approach us saying how "delicious" Alexa was and that they couldn't help but notice her eyes. Because I was at the hospital performing complex surgeries while also moonlighting at outside practices to earn extra money and refine my surgical skills, LeAnn and Alexa became especially close. At times, it must have seemed as if it was just the two of them.

In an effort to stay connected with my growing family during this demanding time, I'd take LeAnn and Alexa in tow with me on weekends when I was covering trauma calls at Mayo Clinic satellite hospitals. To entertain ourselves when I wasn't on call, we would frequently travel to Minneapolis, which has the amazing Mall of America—one of the largest malls in the world.

Unfortunately, even when we tried to go out on family excursions, I was so sleep-deprived that I found it almost impossible to stay awake during the ninety-minute drive from Rochester to Minneapolis, often with poor visibility and treacherously frozen roads. If I didn't watch it, *we'd* wind up in a hospital!

"You're going to kill us!" said LeAnn, often raising her voice to keep me awake. But no matter how hard I tried, I just couldn't keep my eyes open. I had begun battling this excessive sleepiness during medical school. Later, during my residency, I had fallen asleep several times while driving and even crashed into the back of a car once! On the fifteen-minute drive from my home to the hospital, I had driven off the road on numerous occasions. Although I was aware of the condition called *obstructive sleep apnea* with similar symptoms, I always attributed my symptoms to my workload and lack of sleep. However, it was even happening on vacation and on the weekends when I had adequate sleep.

Now that I had a wife and baby girl in the car, I was obviously responsible for much more than just myself, so I had to definitely find out if I had I sleep apnea or not. As LeAnn reminded me, since I now worked at one of the top hospitals in the world, I should take advantage to undergo a proper evaluation at the Mayo Clinic to determine the source of my excessive sleepiness. I did it immediately upon her suggestion, and the sleep study confirmed a diagnosis of obstructive sleep apnea. The results indicated I woke up thirty-two times per hour!

I was given two choices for treatment: use a rather cumbersome CPAP machine or an orthodontic appliance that you simply insert at night, which shifts your lower jaw forward to decrease the chance that your airway closes when you sleep. Knowing that I wanted to be deployable when I returned to Wilford Hall and that the CPAP would make that impossible, I opted for the orthodontic solution—but that turned out to be intolerable. I tried it for three months, but I experienced severe spasms of my jaw muscles that resulted in excruciating pain and terrible temporal headaches. As a result, I had to switch to the CPAP machine, which immediately improved the quality of my sleep and led to much-improved energy levels the following day.

Although my sleep quality and energy levels improved, I was left with the question about how I could be deployable while also in nightly need of this machine. With this in mind, my fellowship director prompted me to schedule a consultation at Wilford Hall. I met with a pulmonologist who told me that I would be nondeployable. When I broke this news to the deputy chairman of the department of orthopaedic surgery at Wilford Hall, all hell broke loose. The deputy believed that I had fabricated the diagnosis to avoid deployment, and he then took his false allegations to the chairman of the department. The chairman at the time was a self-righteous, judgmental Christian who assumed there was a plot in what I had done, which was nothing more than getting the medical help I needed and being honest about it! Talk about a tempest in a teapot and the petty politics involved at a hospital.

I thought I had done the right thing in giving everyone a heads-up about my change in circumstances, which was out of my control. The chairman then notified the pulmonology physician I'd seen that I was lying to avoid deployment. How ridiculous! I had never shirked responsibility or cheated in my entire life. In fact, I had always assumed *additional* responsibilities. However, for some strange reason, they never gave me a chance and ignored the fact that the world-renowned Mayo Clinic would never fabricate a sleep study and give me a fake diagnosis.

It was absurd to even suggest that, but rumors spread throughout the hospital. The chairman and deputy chairman threatened to reassign me to another base. This really worried me, because I knew that if I did not return to Wilford, I would lose the possibility of becoming the chief of spine surgery for the Air Force. Worse still, if I was reassigned to a smaller base, it was likely I wouldn't perform spine surgeries at all. Luckily, despite their attempt to reroute me, the higher-ups who determine Air Force assignments ultimately sent me to Wilford Hall after all. The beauty of that decision was that I would be returning to my hometown of San Antonio, where my family lived and I could have a full-fledged, busy spine position at a busy hospital. I was elated about the assignment, but my chairman and deputy chairman were committed to making me miserable—as I would soon find out.

Chapter Seven

The Hornet's Nest

In July of 2004, with my newly tainted reputation, I returned to Wilford Hall from my fellowship at the Mayo Clinic into what seemed to be a hornet's nest. It was a highly politicized atmosphere, with many of the staff at each other's throats, all related to the heavy deployment tempo.

I decided that I would resume wearing the orthodontic appliance instead of the CPAP machine to treat my sleep apnea. Although it gave me headaches and jaw pain, I figured it was worth it to show I was a team player who was willing to sacrifice like the others. I would pay for that decision later.

It wasn't very long after my arrival at the hospital that the chairman wanted to deploy me into active combat conditions. I was initially scheduled for deployment within just two months of arriving back at Wilford Hall. But in the fall of that year during combat training with our helmet and body armor, I sustained a large herniated disc in my cervical spine, which delayed my deployment until the winter of 2006.

The severe pain I felt in my neck ran all the way down into my left arm. In fact, I could not lift my wrist—though I was still able to perform surgery. However, because my arm was so weak, it was not safe for me to be deployed. I was told that I had to heal for at least a year.

Meanwhile, as the new chief of spine surgery for the Air Force, I was at a definite disadvantage, as I had no surgeon senior to me to whom I could turn in order to discuss complex procedures in the OR. At the Mayo Clinic, there were always several staff surgeons from different disciplines scrubbed in to surgery together to assist one another; but in the Air Force, I didn't have that luxury. I was forced to operate on complex conditions with just a physician assistant and/or a resident.

Nonetheless, I never turned away a case. I felt that it was my responsibility to use my training wisely so that I could help as many people as possible. In fact, my very first case at Wilford Hall turned out to be one of my most challenging cases to date. The patient was an active-duty senior-ranking sergeant suffering from a highly aggressive cancer of the thoracic spine. He had a malignant growth that had penetrated the bone and invaded the spinal canal, threatening to damage the spinal cord, which could lead to paralysis. In addition, both the cancer and the complex surgery necessary to treat it were life-threatening. Unfortunately, the surgery was commonly performed at the Mayo Clinic but rarely tackled at Wilford Hall. After consulting with my lifelong mentor, Dr. Yaszemski, my surgical plan was all set. It was going to be a very delicate surgery, a thirty-hour procedure performed over two days with fifteen hours each day. While I was nervous, I felt confident that I could do it.

In addition to the challenge of stabilizing the spine and removing the tumor without paralyzing the patient, I had to avoid cutting into the tumor, as this would likely result in metastasis and certain death. The case was a resounding success! The surgery required me to remove one half of five vertebral bones in the front, five ribs, and the back half of the spinal bones and muscle in a wide margin around the cancer to avoid spreading it throughout the body. Luckily, there was a cardiothoracic surgeon who helped with the rib excision and a microsurgeon who helped move the back muscle from the other side to cover the defect. I replaced the missing bone with a long metallic cage and bone graft and stabilized the spine over ten levels with titanium screws and rods. Not only was the patient's cancer successfully removed, but his fusion healed solidly, and he is still alive to this day.

The positive outcome of this case, though incredibly stressful, gave me the confidence that I could do anything. It also reinforced my conviction that the quality of my training at the Mayo Clinic had made all the difference. In fact, since that case, I have never turned away any surgery because it was complex or challenging.

However, my colleagues at the hospital were not always so industrious, for a few different reasons. First, since the physicians were working in a military hospital with a fixed salary (rather than in private practice), there was no financial incentive to work harder. No matter how many surgeries they performed, their pay would remain the same. Additionally, military surgeons make 25 percent of the salary of their civilian counterparts. Many of them felt no need to work themselves to the bone for such a meager income. Second, there was a lot of stress related to the looming threat of being deployed, while at the same time, those returning home *after* deployment were exhausted and wanted to work as little as possible in order to recuperate and spend time with their families. Moreover, they didn't have the responsibility of paying practice overhead, since they were employees. Regardless of what my colleagues did, I continued to work long hours while back home, as my prime motivation was to hone my skills as a surgeon and help as many people as I could.

Because the majority of the staff in the hospital were deployed, the surgeons left behind had limited OR time. Because of this, the commander allowed physicians like me time to moonlight off base to ensure proficiency. So, during the two-year period when I was recovering from my disc herniation (before being deployed), I began working off base. Previously, I moonlit as a flight surgeon, but this time it would be as a spine surgeon. Off-duty employment was very strictly controlled: Only sixteen hours per week were allotted to work off base. Those hours had to be performed on weekdays after 5:00 p.m. or on weekends and holidays. We could also take vacation days to moonlight, which I often did (as I was not one to vacation much anyway).

For my first moonlighting gig as a spine surgeon in 2004, I worked with an orthopaedic surgeon in downtown San Antonio who ran a rather a hectic clinic. There were five examination rooms that were always filled with *his* patients (who got priority), leaving me sitting there all day long despite only having a few patients to see. I found it inconsiderate and unsustainable. I looked for a better opportunity shortly after starting.

I was next referred to an elderly orthopaedic surgeon, Dr. Walt Simmons, a southern "gentleman" who had developed his own spinal hardware system for surgery. We agreed that I would get 65 percent of the collections of payment for my patients, and he would take 35 percent for his overhead—which seemed fair to me. Because I was unknown in the area as a surgeon, I hired a marketer for $1,000 a month. As things turned out, the referrals were primarily workers' compensation patients, some of whom had endured up to twelve failed surgeries prior to seeing me. Many of them had undergone years of treatment with poor outcomes. The number of these failed surgeries was shocking! By the time these patients came to me, they were miserable. They were walking around like zombies, sedated by narcotics and worn down by lack of sleep due to the pain. It made me want to give everything I had in order to help them out of their dire situation.

I had always been empathetic in this way toward patients (even when some of my colleagues were not); I truly felt their suffering and wondered how this could happen so often. Thanks to my training at Mayo, I was extremely adept at performing these kinds of revision operations and always accepted those patients right away. However, I did not expect the negative backlash from disgruntled doctors who heard that I was the one who was correcting their work. They spread lies that I performed "excessive surgeries," which was not the case.

I found it ironic that surgeons who had performed multiple failed surgeries on their patients, one level at a time, were suggesting my single surgery was excessive because I fixed all the levels that were abnormal at once. The true measure of the correct diagnosis and surgical plan is defined by the outcome. Some surgeons think the smaller the surgery, the better, even when the symptoms fail to improve. They just keep "spot welding" the spine over and over while failing to alleviate symptoms. Numerous small, unsuccessful surgeries is what I define as excessive, not one surgery that relieves the symptoms. I'm not sure if they understand what "excessive" really means. Understanding what surgery to perform and having the symptoms relieved is not as easy as it seems. A lot of that boils down to where a surgeon trained and how willing they are to be careful and meticulous to ensure the surgery is a success.

When I perform any surgery, revision or otherwise, the only thing I'm thinking about is helping that patient get out of pain with one surgery. I put my heart and soul into their operations. Nothing else matters. Ultimately, I know God is the real healer, so I sincerely devote myself to serving Him and thereby my patients. When they improve, I always give the glory to God, giving credit where credit is due.

For six months, I moonlit at the clinic and performed multiple surgeries (while also paying for my own marketing). The owner of the practice, all the while, kept telling me that he was in the hole and that he would pay me during the "next" pay period. After working Saturdays, Sundays, holidays, and every Monday for six months, I had burned through one-third of my vacation days and had still made no money for my efforts. If there was any doubt about my leaving the practice, LeAnn, who is no-nonsense and has a strong sense of justice, laid down the law: "You either have to demand the payment or leave, but you can't continue to work for free."

As with most things, my time in Simmons's clinic was not all bad. It led to my meeting and befriending his new nurse practitioner, a brilliant guy named Eloy Castaneda. Eloy and I hit it off immediately. He had a lot of experience after working for sixteen years in spinal procedures with two other spine surgeons prior to arriving at this clinic. During my tenure there, Eloy had observed that while my patients were returning without pain, Simmons's patients had infection after infection. Many were also left with nerve injuries after their procedures.

One day, Eloy asked me why my patients were doing so well after spinal surgery. He told me that Simmons had a large number of patients with "unwarranted complications, including infections and nerve injuries, amounting to failed surgeries." In his own words, Eloy shared with me that, in the new practice, he felt like he was "sending his patients off to slaughter" when I wasn't doing their surgery. In order to help Eloy work up his patients so that Simmons could at least have all the information he needed to make the right surgical decision, I outlined in detail my algorithms for evaluating patients: which symptoms led to which tests and which results led to which treatments.

As I've been told by many patients, a lot of surgeons order an MRI and possibly never even look at the images but only read the report when deciding which surgery is necessary. I find this limited evaluation preoperatively leads to failed surgeries. There are several studies and tests necessary to identify the source or sources of pain in order to adequately determine the appropriate surgical intervention necessary to optimize the chance of recovery.

Eloy was eager to attain a deeper understanding of the spine, and he soaked up all that I taught him about the spine over the course of several months. He had a mind like a steel trap. He memorized my algorithms better than most of the people I had trained previously, including some orthopaedic residents. When I decided to leave the "no-pay" clinic at the six-month mark, Eloy had also contemplated leaving, as he felt partially responsible for the surgical failures of Simmons and was concerned over what he also perceived was a lack of ethics. We commiserated about how difficult it was to find someone who truly cared about the patients the way we did.

At first, Eloy and I had committed to one another that we would never add any other practitioners to our practice. We would keep it small. We had both been jaded by our experiences with other doctors in the past who were careless, and we didn't really trust anybody to deliver the kind of care we prided ourselves on—caring for people like they were members of our own family.

After consulting with LeAnn, we decided the only solution was for me to open up my own practice—though I had several obstacles to overcome. First, we had no money. Second, the Air Force had a strict policy against an active-duty serviceman establishing a solo private practice. After reading the rules carefully, I realized a "group" practice would meet the criteria. This alliance with other physicians was crucial. It would allow me the best of both worlds: following the guidelines in the Air Force while remaining able to make extra income in a private group practice. Our new group was technically compliant with the rules and also gave me physician back-up when I was away performing military duties.

The group consisted of a local orthopaedic surgeon, a pain specialist, and Eloy as our nurse practitioner, the primary provider for initial evaluations.

We called the practice The Spine and Orthopaedic Institute, which clashed in name with a different practice locally. They had a building with a similar name although their practice was named very differently. They sued, we counter-sued, and we proved that you can't reserve a generic name. However, to avoid confusion and conflict, we ultimately changed our name to The Orthopaedic & Spine Institute.

Since I was just a military guy with no money, we opened the practice in a bare-bones office—a 2,400-square-foot space with borrowed furniture located in a rundown building in the middle of downtown San Antonio. The quality of our care overshadowed the modesty of the décor.

The start-up went very well, with me doing surgeries on Saturdays and Sundays and on holidays too. As the practice found its rhythm, Eloy remained my right-hand man, a guy with a brilliant memory who effortlessly absorbed all the very complicated algorithms that I learned at Mayo related to patient care for spine patients. He would do the initial intake patient workups, referring them to our team for conservative treatment. If those treatments did not work, then he would send these patients to a surgical consult with me. Through it all, Eloy was absolutely indispensable; he was our anchor, making sure our thriving little practice survived. Frankly, without him, there would have *been* no practice.

Eloy, who was intimidatingly large at 300 pounds, became my biggest cheerleader and best friend; I was more convinced than ever that we could establish a leading spinal practice statewide. Although he was passionate and incredibly empathetic to our patients in need, Eloy was also very outspoken and often said derogatory things about the surgeons whose patients had poor outcomes and came to me for a revision surgery. He was advocating for me, but he was also criticizing other surgeons, which wasn't politically correct. I cautioned him constantly about being careful with this criticisms, but he couldn't help himself.

Eloy had a personality that was larger than life: his crude sense of humor was often punctuated by uproarious laughter. Despite that, he was warm and loving to our patients, though at times he was short-tempered too. It was very difficult to control his behavior. Because we were as close as brothers, I counseled him about toning down what he said in the operating room, especially when it came to criticizing other surgeons. Because he was associated with me, at times, I was given "credit" for his comments, even though they weren't mine. And because of it, I started to gain a few enemies off base in the pain management and spine surgery world.

They already didn't like the fact that a military doctor was treading on their turf; to them, I was a young "punk" who was correcting their surgeries and criticizing them openly (which I wasn't!). All surgeons are human and sometimes either make mistakes or have patients who do not obtain the surgical result we hope for. In any case, though Eloy was fueling the fire with his critical comments, I stayed loyal to him because he had amazing strengths and a kind heart. After all, he was also a superb clinician who made it possible for my practice to stay open while I was active duty. I owed him for his loyalty. I just had to keep working on his delivery.

Meanwhile, on base the word spread about the success of my new practice, as did the predictable resentment about it. While I may have been elated with the booming practice, not everybody was. Predictably, there was a lot of jealousy and animosity on base, which impacted the way I was being treated. Both my chairman of orthopaedics at that time (who was a self-professed Christian and very pious) and his deputy chairman became the antagonists in my military life. They seemed to really resent the fact that I was doing well in the group practice. The environment they created was definitely toxic.

These two guys were hardly setting a good example. Other staff who were violating moonlighting rules by covering trauma calls in three different cities (and states) at once were also openly critical about my moonlighting. I think they were all trying to deflect attention from their questionable practices by pointing the finger at my moonlighting setup—a pretty common tactic!

The irony was that I worked extremely hard on base—longer hours than almost anybody else in my department, which is sort of the nature of spine surgery: big cases, long hours. There were marathon days when I would be in surgery with elective cases until midnight because I wanted to help everybody who came to me. Most surgeons would refer complicated (troublesome to them) cases to another facility, like Georgetown or Mayo. But I didn't turn *anyone* away, feeling that it was my responsibility to take care of those patients in pain. I always worried about their outcomes if they sought out the wrong treatment. The last thing I wanted to do was say, "You need to go off base to seek care." That just wasn't the way I thought.

There I was, working all these extra hours *on base* while being persecuted for my success *off base*. However, I should not have been surprised, because the military is basically a socialist environment. If you don't march exactly the same way they do, you're an outlier. I've never been an inside-the-box, black-and-white kind of thinker. I think in a creative, artistic way. That's one reason I can adapt to perform complicated revision surgeries that other people aren't interested in handling. I think about the science *and* the art of medicine. But that kind of thinking doesn't fit into the typical military environment. So, even though I got letters of commendation all the time from the general for consistently positive patient outcomes, I was still a bit of an outcast. Part of it was the way that I chose to moonlight by starting a practice versus covering trauma calls like everyone else. Another differentiating factor was that I didn't attend college at the Air Force Academy, making me different than many of my colleagues.

Many in my department surmised that money was the sole motivator. Isn't that what everyone assumes about successful surgeons and doctors? I find it a strange double standard that entertainers, athletes, Wall Streeters, and personal injury attorneys make tens and hundreds of millions without issue, but when a hardworking doctor does well, I've noticed that some people—even fellow doctors—resent it. It's as if all those years of medical school, then working 100 hours a week while assuming tremendous responsibility for someone's life, doesn't deserve a high income. I'll never understand that perspective. I have no issue with LeBron James, Patrick Mahomes, Tom Cruise, Jeff Bezos, Elon Musk, or Bill Gates making millions or billions of dollars. They generate great value. I believe they're entitled to a portion of that value.

While I held these opinions strongly, I certainly wasn't going to share them in the military, as thinking outside the box was taboo. I would later find out that the chairman who preceded the pious Christian chairman even disapproved of my version of moonlighting, telling me it was "not what the Air Force had envisioned," even though it complied with every rule and restriction. This was a guy I really respected and who liked me as a resident under him.

Not surprisingly, Simmons, the doctor whose practice Eloy and I left, filed a complaint against me with my commander, suggesting that *I* had cheated him and had set up an illegal practice that violated the military's rules. This was astounding, since it was Simmons who was cheating me out of my deserved fees! But his accusation plays into a familiar theme I'd seen often: the guilty party accuses the innocent once they're exposed and no longer able to take advantage. I think crooks all go to the same class—Deception 101: Smoke and Mirrors.

After reviewing my practice arrangement, the military attorneys (JAG officers) ignored Simmons's complaint; they were impressed by how I had followed the rules, albeit creatively. They felt the formation of an LLC was the correct way to moonlight while protecting the physician and the Air Force from liability. They suggested

I give a talk to other physicians on how to safely set up a practice within the rules of the military. But as my practice blossomed off base, this entire issue became a sore spot to the colleagues who continued to resent my outside-the-box approach to moonlighting.

It wasn't long before our new practice really caught on, booking back-to-back appointments with multiple patients in need of revision surgeries. Beyond their trusting my years of training at Mayo and in the Air Force, you might be wondering why they were coming to me when there were many spinal surgeons in the area. Interestingly, back then in San Antonio, no one would touch another doctor's post-surgical patient!

In fact, there was kind of an unwritten political rule that if one physician had performed a surgery (even if it failed) no other specialist would second-guess that doctor, much less take on the patient. I guess they either wanted to avoid the complexity of a revision surgery or avoid ruffling any other surgeon's feathers by "fixing" their failures. This left a niche open for me.

So, when case managers (usually nurses) at workers' compensation found out that I was willing to treat patients with failed surgeries, my practice blew up. In record numbers, these patients would recover and return to work. No one had ever seen these kinds of recovery before, so our practice became very successful. In fact, we had 90 percent growth every year for the first five years, even though I was still on active duty and only able to work after hours on Saturday, Sunday, holidays, and one weeknight a week. The practice was able to bring in substantial revenue that allowed us to feel incredibly hopeful about the future.

From the start, one secret to the success of our group practice was finding a hospital that would allow me to perform elective surgeries on weekends, which was atypical for any hospital unless the surgery was an emergency procedure.

Fortuitously, in 2005, I was approached by a small privately owned off-base hospital in San Antonio called Innova. Their representative told me that their facility could accommodate me and offer their surgical facilities any day of the week, including Saturdays, Sundays, after hours, and holidays. It was the perfect solution, and once I began performing small procedures there, I was amazed at the level of care and the compassion demonstrated by the nursing and administrative staff. It reminded me of what I had experienced at the Mayo Clinic. As time passed, I started doing more and more complicated surgeries there.

Over time, once we settled in, my vascular surgeon and anesthesiologist agreed we could expand the complexity and the number of the cases we were performing, which included anterior/posterior fusions of the spine. Not only were our patients doing remarkably well, but the hospital began to really thrive due to the volume of spinal procedures we were bringing in.

In fact, even though I was only a part-time surgeon at Innova, the hospital was making significant revenue from my operations, so they offered me a percentage share in the hospital itself. It was an intriguing proposal, but I didn't have any reserve money to invest. I was still active duty. There was no way I could buy into the hospital at that point, though all that would later change. The idea of having partial ownership in a hospital is very attractive to many surgeons. We expect that our ownership will bring with it some control over the quality of care being provided, input into the patient experience and the hiring of staff, and maybe even some profit outside the ever-decreasing reimbursements from the government and insurance. Hospital owners know this, and many of them use it to take advantage of idealistic and unsuspecting physicians. It's a way to capture a surgeon's patient volume and increase the hospital's revenue.

Although it can be an ideal scenario that leads to increased patient satisfaction and doctor-directed care resulting in less complications, ownership doesn't work well in many cases. Many of these owners use the physician buy-in to lock physicians into a real estate deal where the general partners (not the physicians) flip the real estate to a venture capitalist group or real estate investment trust (REIT) with an immediate upside for them. That flip increases the overhead for the operating group the physicians own part of, thus decreasing or eliminating the profits altogether. It's a little bit of a scam.

This opportunity became nearly impossible with the passage of the Affordable Care Act in 2010, which completely eliminated a physician's ability to buy into a hospital that does government business. So, as it stands, physicians can only own up to 40 percent of a hospital—and only one with private insurance cases, further shifting the control and profit to the businessmen and away from physicians.

Chapter Eight

Workers' *De*compensation

At the same time my group practice was thriving, there were stressors happening on the home front. When I returned from Mayo in 2004, I began noticing that my father was losing his train of thought mid-sentence. It took a year of convincing him to finally consent to a CT scan, which revealed severe atrophy of the frontal and temporal regions of his brain. In other words, he was suffering from dementia. We all felt terrible for him. After all, throughout his entire life, Dad's strongest asset had been his mind, which was now literally wasting away. Worse yet, there was no treatment to slow the progression of the disease.

In the earliest stages, he was aware of what he would be facing. It was sadly ironic that in his practice as a psychologist, he had focused on the care of nursing-home patients, many of whom *had* dementia. Because he was an expert in this field, getting the disease himself was like a dagger to the heart. He was only fifty-nine years old at the time. In a flash, he could no longer practice. And sadly, he had not financially prepared for retirement, much less for an unexpected diagnosis like this. His Air Force pension was minimal, and because he had not saved much money, my parents began to really struggle.

In fact, one of my strongest motivations to moonlight was to help them financially. One of my sweetest memories of my father before he lost all cognition was how much he loved our daughter Alexa, who was just two years old at the time he got sick. He was so sweet and loving to her. Watching them together was a true joy. Although Alexa, a momma's girl, wouldn't usually let anyone hold her except LeAnn, she loved her Papa and let him hold her all the time.

Over the next fourteen years, it was grueling to watch such a brilliant man suffer from the progressive destruction of his mind and his body. It's tragic to witness this withering process, as someone gradually slips into a vegetative state. During his last five years, he couldn't communicate or feed himself. When he finally passed away in May 2018, I think we all breathed a sigh of relief for him because we knew his suffering had ended and that he was at home, finally in Heaven.

In 2005, just at the time I began the group practice, LeAnn and I had our second child, a son named Caden. He was the chubbiest, cutest baby I had ever seen in my life. Unlike Alexa, he was a daddy's boy and would never let me put him down. He was the first to run excitedly to greet me every time I came home, and he would break my heart every time I left in the morning to go to work, always standing in the window bawling as I drove away. He seemed to have a special attachment to me and was always waiting to be snuggled and hugged. It felt so great when his eyes lit up when he saw me.

As the years went by, Caden became one of the most charismatic and charming kids I had ever met. Even adults would come up to meet us, wondering who his parents were, as he was so friendly and polite. Later he became a whiz academically, excelling in school with little effort. He was naturally entrepreneurial and always saved up all the money he got for holidays and birthdays; he was blessed with a business mind unlike any kid I'd ever met. At nine years old—without any prompting—he started an exclusive sneaker business, purchasing and reselling high-end athletic shoes, making $40,000 a year. No doubt, LeAnn and I believe that his business prowess will only continue to grow with age and experience.

At this point, I was in my second year as a staff surgeon and professor of spine surgery at Wilford Hall. In addition to my responsibilities as an officer and surgeon, I stayed busy training residents, medical students, and physician assistant fellows, all in the orthopaedic department. In addition, of course, my off-base practice was thriving. Still, I didn't want my children growing up like I had, rarely seeing their father. So even though it was a challenge to maintain balance, I made sure I spent every free minute at home with my family.

That all changed in October 2006. There we were—in the middle of Operation Enduring Freedom, the official name used by the U.S. government for the global war on terrorism. This was the moment when I was thrown into a war zone for the first time as a combat surgeon, leaving behind the group practice in the capable hands of Eloy with our other physicians.

Although I thought I was prepared for this kind of assignment, I wasn't. Nobody could be. What I saw on the field shocked me.

There were extremity injuries of every variety from bombs, shrapnel, and bullets.

It was nonstop horror; it was worse trauma than in any Level I trauma center in America. No injury was simple, with entire bodies blown up and simultaneously burned because the insurgents laced the bombs with diesel fuel. Many times, soldiers would come in with multiple extremities blown off. It was horrendous. The sheer number of people suffering was beyond anything I had ever seen.

Our operating rooms were a labyrinth of connected military tents. When it was hot outside, it was even hotter inside. When it was cold, we were freezing. When it rained, there were puddles of water on the makeshift floor. In summer, there were so many flies in the tent that the flypaper hanging from the ceiling wasn't even visible.

As officers, we had small trailers that were adjacent to the C-RAM (counter rocket, artillery, and mortar) gun, which precisely shot the enemy mortars out of the sky. It went off all night long. It was amazing to see, but the noise of it made it impossible to sleep. To distract ourselves, there was really nothing to do other than to watch reruns of TV series while snacking on dried mangoes and pub mix. When we weren't doing trauma surgery, this was our nighttime entertainment.

To handle the tremendous volume of injured patients, we had a team of four orthopaedic surgeons and two PAs who took care of all the orthopaedic injuries to the arms, legs, and spine. We sometimes had up to forty-five patients at a time, one right after another. And because nearly every patient was experiencing multisystem injuries, we functioned like a giant trauma team, with multiple surgeons from different disciplines, technicians, nurses, and PAs all working around the clock, synchronizing their efforts.

Right on the field, medics would descend on patients who were literally on the brink of death, making instant assessments that provided lifesaving interventions. Military helicopters would then transport the gravely injured patients to our in-theater hospital for further treatment. Despite the severity of these injuries, our highly skilled teams worked tirelessly to save life and limb. War-injured servicemen had a 90 percent survival rate *if* they made it to our hospital. I can proudly say that we saved almost everybody. It was amazing. Over the course of four and a half months in 2006, our orthopaedic team alone performed 780 major surgeries!

The base was being bombed constantly, so much so that we jokingly called it Mortar-rita-ville. We would receive incoming notifications ten to twelve times a day of incoming mortars. Through it all, I never worried about getting killed or blown up. I never suffered from post-traumatic stress disorder because I was able to compartmentalize my experience while there. I focused on the patients and their injuries and left it all in the operating room. It's the only way to prevent the emotional burden from creeping into your psyche.

During this first deployment to Iraq in 2006, though my life was in danger at times, I was much more worried about how my family was coping without me back home. In my absence, LeAnn, who was always super-organized, was single-handedly managing all operations as the official CFO and COO of our practice—all the while raising two small children. She maintained the budget and ensured that the business side of the practice was run correctly. All this placed an extreme amount of stress on her as she attempted to balance motherhood and the practice.

Every night, I would call to check in, and Alexa would promptly answer and pass the phone to LeAnn saying, "Mommy misses you. Talk to mommy." Even at four years old, she was an incredibly observant child with amazing sensitivity and intuition. Maybe that's why she adored my father so much, seeing past his infirmities to his kindheartedness.

After being away for five months, when I finally returned home, I felt a huge sense of relief and happiness. There's no greater sense of exhilaration than being reunited with your family after an extended period of time. When I first saw LeAnn and the kids and all our friends and relatives waiting for me in the airport, I broke down in tears and just hugged them for as long as I could. We were all overjoyed.

As I looked at LeAnn, I was concerned. I could see she had lost at least twenty pounds, even though she was at a healthy weight before I left. The stress had certainly taken its toll. Something had changed in Alexa too. Prior to my deployment, as I said, she had more or less ignored me ever since she was born, shrugging off my repeated attempts to hug and kiss her. But suddenly she was very affectionate. I was thrilled.

The adjustment back to life in San Antonio with the family was rapid. My time in Iraq had been occupied by two things: doing surgery and working out. In fact, our team of orthopaedic specialists in Iraq did everything together, including exercise, so we had all improved our physical fitness to an extreme. I was now in peak condition, just as fit as I was while playing football in college.

I expected my return from my first deployment to be the proof to everyone at Wilford Hall that I was truly a team player, but some of them continued to behave strangely, having always doubted my sleep apnea diagnosis, which could have prevented my deployment. My choosing to deploy regardless should have been evidence that I would never shirk my duty, but in order to deploy, I had started to wear an orthodontic appliance instead of using my CPAP machine. As I mentioned earlier, this appliance came with consequences. It shifted my jaw forward and to the left, resulting in a crossbite. I thought my military colleagues on base would commend me on my willingness to sacrifice to this extent in order to deploy, but they did not. I don't even know why I actually cared what they thought, but I hated the fact that they considered me dishonest. Later, to solve the sleep apnea issue once and for all, I opted to have a rather painful surgery that removed a portion of the soft palate and tonsils, along with radio-frequency burning/shrinking of the base of the tongue. The goal was to decrease the soft tissue bulk that relaxes, blocking the airway when one sleeps. I was also forced to get braces for a second time to correct my jaw alignment.

No matter what I did, how well my patients did, or how hard I worked, I still felt like an outsider at Wilford Hall. To make matters worse, there still remained controversy (and jealousy) when it came to my moonlighting work at my clinic. I got to the point where I distanced myself from the staff surgeons in the department and just focused on the residents and my patients.

Upon getting back into the routine in February of 2007 both at Wilford Hall and my clinic, I could feel the difference as a surgeon. My previous deployment to Iraq in 2006 had honed my skills and enhanced my sense of confidence and steadiness under pressure.

Meanwhile, in terms of private practice, our little office was about to get a major upgrade. An orthopaedic surgeon I had known in the military, Rich Steffen, reached out to me about the possibility of relocating my practice to a new building that he and his team of six doctors had just built. It was a state-of-the-art compound located right next to the San Antonio Spurs training facility. The building seemed perfect, seeing as Rich and his staff were the team doctors for the San Antonio Spurs. His group of orthopaedic sports surgeons also took care of many of the high school and college athletes in the city. Fortunately for me, they were looking for a spine surgeon to occupy space in the building and round out their specialties, although I wasn't joining their practice—just relocating my clinic to their location.

The allure of being the spine surgeon for the Spurs really piqued my interest. I accepted the offer to relocate and constructed a 3,500-square-foot clinic space—a real upgrade from where we had come, with a price tag to match. Our overhead dramatically skyrocketed as we finished out the interior decor. Around this time, I was approached by one of my colleagues on base, an Army hand surgeon named Joel Nilsson, who asked if he could join our practice too. Joel and I had become very close friends during our deployment to Iraq. And, like me, he was a strong Christian who had great integrity. He was also planning to eventually separate from the military but wanted to stay in San Antonio. It was a perfect match. Eloy and I would focus on complex spinal surgeries, while Joel would manage the general orthopaedic patients.

At the Texas Center for Athletes, I was now the official "Spine Surgeon for the Spurs," or so I thought. I quickly discovered that my recruitment was merely an effort to fill their medical office building with yet another high-paying tenant, with no real plan to refer the Spurs players (or *any* patients) to me! In fact, the sports group also hired sports medicine doctors who were not surgeons or orthopaedic specialists. They were the ones who provided the majority of the care, and they rarely referred patients out.

To add insult to injury, I was promised that our practice's name would be placed on the outside of the building, but that never happened either. And then everything changed when the physician group decided to cash in on their investment and sold their building to a tyrannical REIT based in Boston. In years to come, this would prove to be a major issue for us. REITs don't know their tenants. It is just a group of individuals who invest in real estate. Obviously, the bottom line is profit and asset-building. That's not always a bad thing, but for us it was. I should have been a lot more suspicious of their intentions when they requested new contracts tying all the clinic space together into one agreement. We had individual lease agreements for each space but they wanted them connected. I did not think it was a big deal. But it was because it meant if you defaulted on one clinic, you defaulted on them all. I should have had a real estate attorney review the lease and amend it to protect my interests, but I didn't...big mistake.

Despite these challenges, we were thriving. I was repeatedly approached by former military doctors who wanted to join my practice due to our obvious success. My hope was that we could create a one-stop shop for all our patients, with multiple specialists available to address any issue.

Conversely, my department was a mess at Wilford Hall. Our chairman, who few of us respected, left the military in 2008 and was replaced by the deputy chairman, a Napoleonic surgeon whose personality was even more insufferable. He was neither a nice guy nor a good surgeon. The chairman who left was the man who tried to turn everyone against me when he thought I was lying about having sleep apnea upon my return to Wilford Hall from my fellowship. However, prior to his leaving, he did say something that has stuck with me to this day. He was a devout Christian like me.

The main difference was he talked a good game, but his actions rarely followed. After all the issues I had faced in the military—the attempted blackballing from the orthopaedic residency by the previous chairman, the attempt to block me from a spine fellowship by the two prior spine staff surgeons, prior investigations—he couldn't help but acknowledge that every attempt to attack me had failed miserably (including his own). Prior to leaving the Air Force he told me, "You must live a good life because God always seems to protect you." His comment made me think of the story of Daniel in the Bible. I did feel like I had been unfairly targeted for so long, but God shielded me from every attack. I was so ready to leave the Air Force because of all I had gone through. I had no idea what was coming next.

Meanwhile, the repeated deployments to Iraq took an enormous toll on the hospital staffing. In fact, 75 percent of our staff had been deployed at one time or another to either Iraq or Afghanistan. This made it exceedingly difficult to perform surgery back home at Wilford Hall, where we were relegated to one day per week of surgery.

There was no way a surgeon could maintain proficiency, let alone improve skills, with this paltry allowance of time—especially when the staff left at 3:00 p.m. It was socialized medicine at its worst.

At that time, my junior spine partner, who seemed more interested in golfing than in doing surgery, claimed *I* wasn't invested in the military. Meanwhile, I was using both his operating room time and mine, performing complicated surgeries as often as possible. But I was still limited by the restriction on hours per day, so as much as I wanted to be busy with surgeries, this situation was untenable. Although it was far from ideal, I used as many hours as were available to me to continue to grow as a surgeon. I was constantly looking for the perfect opportunity to increase my surgical volume and knowledge by moonlighting.

I had observed many surgeons help companies design spinal implants. In fact, several of my mentors had implants on the market that were very popular amongst spine surgeons. I wanted to do the same. Many times, companies employ engineers who created theoretically good devices that fall flat when they are used for patient care because engineers have no practical experience. Surgeons can really help to innovate and improve care by consulting with companies to design new and improved products for patients that actually work.

So, in 2008, part of my moonlighting duties included consulting with a new U.S. device manufacturer called Allure. The company was owned by a seasoned medical products professional, Julia Eller, who was the previous COO of Altiva and AcroMed, both successful spinal implant companies. When those companies closed, she created Allure. I began consulting with Allure to improve the consistency and shape of bone graft and metallic implants used in spine surgeries.

In an effort to improve what was then available for spine surgery, I had invented multiple enhancements to the standard designs for spinal screws and plates.* I drew designs for retractors, derotators, and a construct for the back of the head and cervical spine

---

* Years prior, while in my fellowship, without the benefit of an engineer or a patent attorney, I had attempted a so-called "poor man's" patent by mailing the concepts back to *myself*, thinking it would protect my "intellectual property" without any actual patent protections. I had drawn screws with blades that extended from the tip once inserted to increase the hold on the bone; these were screws that had an internal screw that expanded the tip, like a drywall anchor (for soft bone).

with connectors that attached to the screws instead of the rods to improve the strength and functionality of the fixation. I designed plates for the front and sides of the spine to fit between the blood vessels and under the esophagus with compression mechanisms that improved the healing potential of the bone. I worked on changing the handling properties of bone graft so it wouldn't float away when placed on the spine and the dimensions of structural bone graft to improve stability and fusion rates.

Throughout this process, I trusted Julia. We brainstormed for literally hours each day about different designs and implants—conversations we had during my drive to work and on the way home. I won't bore you with details, but basically, we discussed new designs for spinal hardware for the neck, midback, and lower back, along with bone graft designs and even novel ideas about coating implants to prevent infection! It was a full immersion project for me. I sent drawings and detailed descriptions of all my ideas, researched the literature, wrote out detailed surgical technique guides, and created names for my line of products based upon Latin terms. I even created logos and color schemes to make the products appealing.

Through it all, from day one, I consulted with a healthcare attorney to make sure that everything I did in my moonlighting life complied with state, federal, and military regulations.

As a military doctor, I had even more regulations to comply with, even if it did not involve direct patient care. My time moonlighting had to be carefully monitored to avoid going over the allotted hours per week. I couldn't work during the duty day unless I was on leave (vacation) or if it was a federal holiday. I had to maintain commander approval and couldn't be the sole provider of care for any patient. Additionally, as a physician, I had to make sure I was paid for my time based on a fair market value per hour arrangement. This number had to be approved by my healthcare attorney, who also reviewed every contract and even created the majority of the contracts I followed. In fact, he drafted the intellectual property contract between me and Julia's implant company to ensure it followed all the federal and state statutes. He also did compliance reviews regularly and sent a compliance letter confirming the arrangement still complied with the laws. Thank God for that!

Companies frequently offer consulting agreements as a way to coax doctors and surgeons into using their products. In many of these cases, there is no true consulting happening. The products have already been created and are being mass produced, so no real input from doctors is necessary in developing them. Be wary of companies who ask you to review products they have on the market in turn for payment. Stay clear of "consulting agreements" or "intellectual property agreements," in which there is a mere "review of the products used" and no real design input. My healthcare attorney recommended deferring royalty payments on products designed by the surgeon when they are used on his/her patients. That way, there can be no suggestion of impropriety. The company's attorney will not come to your defense if an issue arises. Use your own.

Consulting agreements are very tricky. There have been several physicians and implant companies that have been indicted and penalized for violating the rules that govern such arrangements. Surgeons have to be wary of companies who offer to pay for input into a device or product that is already in use. That is not a true design agreement. The number of hours and work effort has to be clearly documented. Records should reflect exactly what advice and recommendations were provided, along with drawings, and technique guides, etc. Otherwise, these types of consulting agreements can be seen as a way to induce a surgeon to use products in exchange for money, thus, an inducement and violation of the Anti-Kickback laws. Other surgeons have made the poor decision to consult in those types of arrangements only to find themselves federally indicted for kickbacks.

I worked diligently to get my ideas to market but nothing was happening quickly; and there were more important (and concerning) things about to occur in my life.

Just as I was preparing to leave for my second deployment to Iraq in 2009, I discovered that the "southern gentleman"—the doctor whose practice Eloy and I had left years earlier—continued to stir up problems. Failing to implicate me to the military for setting up a group practice, he now filed a new complaint with the Texas Workers' Compensation Commission (TWCC).

Simmons had conveniently befriended the medical director of the TWCC at the time and decided to use that connection to strike back at me for leaving his practice. So began another investigation against me alleging that seven of my cases were performed with poor outcomes and, thus, violated the standard of care. To make matters worse, they alleged the same directly to the Air Force, which was now forced to investigate my outcomes in the military as well. Considering the numerous letters of commendation I had received for amazing patient outcomes from the general who was my hospital commander, I couldn't believe this could ever happen. But the Air Force had to do their "due diligence" to prove everything was kosher with my surgical outcomes.

The strange thing was that every single one of those patients, except one, had returned to full duty without restrictions after a successful surgery. After hearing about the investigation, LeAnn consulted with a spine surgeon turned lawyer who had a similar experience as a doctor for the TWCC.

He freaked her out by telling her that not only was I likely to lose my medical license, but that it would also cost $500,000 to defend me. That was a punch in the gut, and she understandably panicked, especially since I was about to leave for Iraq and we didn't have anywhere close to that amount of money.

With the added stress of leaving my family for a war zone and yet another unfounded investigation, one could imagine that one of the most depressing days of my life was the day I left for my second deployment to Baghdad, in 2009. This time, I knew what I was getting into—risking my life in a country where U.S. servicemen continued to be gravely injured by enemy artillery and bombs. I was leaving behind my wife and kids, who were now six and four, and a civilian practice that was now at full capacity. I knew how emotionally difficult this deployment would be for LeAnn, who also had to worry about the terrifying conversation she had with the doctor turned attorney that I could lose my license. Now she had to worry about this as well as trying to keep the practice afloat while taking care of the kids. The only good thing about this mission was that it was mostly uneventful, as the frequency of mortar rounds had dropped dramatically, and the volume of injuries and mass casualties dropped with it. We were still busy doing surgeries but not nearly at the pace of 2006. Yes, we still performed many complicated procedures, but the decline in volume and the slow withdrawal of our troops made for a much less stressful deployment.

This slower pace of life on the base created an opportunity to optimize fitness. So, once again, my band of orthopaedic cohorts and I exercised faithfully every day. I committed to becoming as healthy and lean as possible and was definitely in the best shape of my life, maybe even surpassing my college football days. It kept my mind off of my worries at home.

Although this second tour in Iraq was slated as a short three-month deployment, the Napoleonic chairman back home at Wilford Hall had the idea to swap my three-month deployment with his six-month deployment. When that failed, he thought to extend my deployment while in Iraq. Luckily, the commander on the ground in Iraq saw through his ploy when a senior-ranking colleague deployed with me explained what was happening behind the scenes. The commander in Iraq put an immediate stop to the shenanigans. As a typical weasel would, the chairman at Wilford Hall then found a way to change everyone's deployment to a shorter three-month interval to avoid deploying for six months himself. Ultimately his selfishness helped the rest of the department to have shorter deployments, which turned out to be a good thing. Once again, God had intervened to protect me from a despot with selfish motives. I was praying He would do the same with the TWCC investigation.

Chapter Nine

The Love of Money

In the summer of 2009, I finally returned home from my last deployment. I was overjoyed to see my family again and relieved to know that I would never need to deploy again. In fact, I was even more excited that my commitment to the military was ending after fourteen years of active service.

But now, it was time to face the Texas Workers' Compensation Commission (TWCC) investigation. Fortunately, I was referred to a great attorney who had previously been the general counsel to the Texas Medical Board, Timothy Weitz. He was a no-nonsense former officer in the U.S. Marines who helped me understand the process thoroughly. After reviewing each case, Tim and his brother, Mark, realized the case was strictly an attempt at retribution from Simmons and his new buddy, the TWCC medical director. After putting all the facts together, the Weitz brothers and I arranged a status conference meeting with the medical director of the TWCC and his team. At the hearing I was totally prepared. They clearly underestimated the depth of my training at Mayo and my understanding of the science of spine surgery. I presented each case followed by letters from each patient confirming their successful recovery and return to work. Even the one case that supposedly resulted in a disability was a fraud, as we had film of her leaving our clinic on a walker, folding it up, and then jogging to her car! The medical director thought he had me stumped on that patient until I played the video. I had proven my point, and the embarrassed medical director—whose mouth was agape through the majority of my case presentations—rushed out of the room at the end, telling my attorney, "Call me when you get a chance." Soon after, he dropped all allegations and the case entirely. In the end, it was evident that I surpassed the standard of care, but my frustrations grew more and more with this politically driven field I had entered.

I never expected any of these things could happen to someone with good patient outcomes. But clearly, that was not the case. I started to realize the system was flawed on so many levels. It was nothing like I expected. There were unscrupulous physicians and even systems, like the TWCC, in which people will do or say *anything* necessary to take all that you had worked to accomplish without justification—even in the illustrious field of medicine.

As you can imagine, this experience left me quite irritated with workers' compensation, a system where necessary surgical care is perpetually denied by doctors who sell out their colleagues and have no regard for patients' well-being, relegating patients to years of failed conservative treatment and often leaving them with permanent nerve damage and lifelong pain and narcotic medication addiction as a result. On the rare occasion surgery would be approved and performed, the workers' compensation insurers would hire a turncoat doctor to retroactively deny the procedure and all the costs associated with it. Think about that. This was after the surgery was *approved* and performed. That boggled my mind! How in the world could that happen?! What a criminal system to allow a doctor who never even saw a patient to deny the surgery *after* it was performed. In what other industry is that even possible? The experience with the TWCC investigation was my final straw.

In 2009 I opted out of the Texas workers' compensation system. And I have not seen a Texas workers' compensation patient ever since. It's unfortunate, but the system is so flawed that it puts both patients and doctors at extreme risk.

That year, I also began looking for other product innovations in spine surgery. By my side during this product development period was my brother, Bryan, who had been in the Air Force as a medic and was hoping to attend medical school after leaving the military. However, he later switched gears to work in the medical industry instead.

Bryan's background in science helped in the research we both conducted to identify novel implant technologies. He actually found a company in Turkey that had patented a process that could coat metallic implants with silver nanoparticles to prevent infection. For two years, we consulted with the designing surgeon in Turkey in conjunction with Julia's implant company in an effort to bring those implants to the United States.

In 2009, I became the U.S. distributor of the silver-coated implants, but the financials were impossible, as they wanted an exorbitant $25 million for the patent rights. Additionally, they were unable to obtain FDA clearance for the silver-coated screw system. Nonetheless, I continued to work on designing different systems of screws, plates, and other implants for the spine with

Julia, still hoping that I could eventually bring my designs to the market.

During this same time, I was promised repeatedly by Julia's company that the designs I had helped conceptualize were in the process of being tested and manufactured, but I never saw any finished products, despite hours of work each month. Retrospectively, I doubt they were ever being made. My efforts to get new implants to market were falling flat.

With the TWCC debacle behind me, I was revving up my side practice once again, discussing with LeAnn strategies for increasing our patient volume. It was in the fall of that year that Innova's director of marketing, John Hall, introduced me to a busy chiropractor named Garry Craighead, who owned four federal workers' compensation clinics in central and south Texas, clearly a good source of potential patients for me. I had no idea what I was in for.

The night I met Dr. Craighead, he came strolling into the restaurant wearing Elton John–style sunglasses in a dimly lit room. He had a jacket made of sequins, like Liberace, and "rock star" hair. As I found out, he actually fancied himself "the rock-star chiropractor" of San Antonio, quite a distinction. Even more unusual were his mannerisms. In conversation, he would frequently flail his arms or legs wildly around in circles as if he were under the influence of drugs and/or alcohol. Was he? I don't know. All I can say is that this was the strangest first meeting with a so-called medical professional! Yet despite his eccentricities, there was something oddly endearing about the guy. He actually seemed very nice.

Despite my initial aversion to Craighead, John Hall assured me that he was a standup guy with a vast stream of patients in and out of his office, many of whom would potentially require surgery, thus increasing my volume of procedures at Innova Hospital. He told me they needed a good surgeon. With this in mind, Innova asked that I see some of Craighead's patients in *his* clinic, even though I was concerned about his seemingly unprofessional demeanor.

Not long after we met, Craighead invited me and LeAnn to his house in Austin for an extravagant Fourth of July party, a celebration that included a fireworks display that looked like a New Year's Eve extravaganza. And while this massive display of wealth was impressive, it was not enticing to me. Nor was the guest list, a jaw-dropping mixture of judges and Department of Labor union leaders, mixed in with local politicians—all of them intermingling with medical personnel. There was something suspect about this mix of local characters and physicians that entirely destroyed the sense of propriety that I imagined all doctors should demonstrate.

That was the night I first met a Russian businessman named Semyon Narosov, who I was told had once been a physical therapist. From the moment I set eyes on him, I did not like this guy at all. I shouldn't have been surprised I met him through Craighead.

Narosov asked me what I did for work, and when I told him that I was a spine surgeon, his only question was quantitative. "How many surgeries can you do in a day?" he inquired as if I were producing sweaters in a factory. Much to his disapproval, I told him that to ensure successful surgical outcomes, I typically performed only one big fusion per day or two smaller surgeries.

He was unimpressed with that number and continued his brash inquisition by saying, "I know surgeons who can perform between five and ten spine surgeries a day!" I found this number staggering and questionable. I suppose anyone can fly through an operation, cutting corners and doing poor-quality work, but there was no way to perform that many surgeries meticulously and wind up with good outcomes. "What drives me," I told him, "is the success of the surgeries, not the number of procedures that I perform nor the income." That conversation ended rather abruptly as I walked away, looking for a more engaging person to talk with.

Tracking back to our initial meeting at the restaurant in 2009, Dr. Craighead had bragged about a thirty-three-year-old entrepreneur from Dallas named Andrew Hillman. Craighead described him as a whiz kid who owned more than sixty businesses in the medical industry, which included partnerships with companies ranging from chiropractic clinics and pharmacies to marketing companies and beyond.

According to Craighead, Hillman was primarily responsible for the success of Forest Park Medical Center in Dallas, then a thriving hospital known by most spine and orthopaedic surgeons as the model physician-owned facility in the Lone Star State due to its financial success and posh facilities.

In our meeting, Craighead called Andrew Hillman on the phone to make an introduction. During that first conversation with Andrew, he seemed affable and fun-loving. He was a little bit of a fast talker and clearly confident in his business abilities to the point of being an obvious braggart. His inflections and mannerisms were a combination of Mark Zuckerberg and Jordan Belfort (the Wolf of Wall Street). He talked about how successful Forest Park was and took a lot of the credit for it. He almost immediately attempted to recruit me to Forest Park to perform part-time surgery on patients there.

However, since I was based in San Antonio, I wasn't very comfortable with the idea of traveling to Dallas on a regular basis.

After all, I didn't know anyone in Dallas that I trusted to see my patients or follow them in my absence. So, I brushed off the idea, though I admit that I found Andrew to be a likable guy.

If nothing else, he was a born salesman, a natural entrepreneur with a rather enticing way of complimenting doctors and befriending them—myself included. And despite his somewhat crude manner and sniveling demeanor (an odd blend of rudeness and manic pattern of speech), his persona made you drop your guard. Little did I know then that virtually everything he did and said was a plan to create an elaborate web of companies that were far more focused on making *him* rich than on improving patients' lives.

I don't mind a motivated businessperson, but I am dogmatic about honesty and integrity. As I would learn, much later, he wasn't anything close to honest. But with Andrew, I tended to trust him, as we seemed to have a common bond. We talked about the commonality between Judaism and Christianity, and he seemed to be equally devoted to his faith, which added another layer of commonality and trust. To add further credibility, he talked nonstop about how his supposed professional motto was now, "Compliance, compliance, compliance." And to prove it, he claimed that he had hired an army of retired federal attorneys and a team of other attorneys to ensure compliance for all of his businesses.

In a conversation that would foreshadow events to come, I remember that he talked to me about how he had once had a run-in with the feds when he was the nineteen-year-old owner of a durable medical equipment company. One of his marketers had been passing out gift cards to physicians who ordered their medical supplies—kickbacks for referrals—which was an illegal practice. (In medicine, it is illegal to trade anything of value for referring patients. This became the case with the passage of the Stark law and Anti-Kickback laws.)

He explained that he was exonerated but that the experience made him even more careful and compliant with the regulations. This prior federal indictment should have been a red flag, but my strong faith sometimes leads me to trusting people more than I should. (My former pastor once told me I err too much toward grace, while LeAnn tends to err too much toward justice.)

I should have stopped right there and had nothing further to do with this guy Andrew, but I decided to give him grace when he told me that he had been exonerated and had "learned his lesson." He certainly seemed both successful and contrite, having surrounded himself with a team of healthcare attorneys to ensure total compliance.

I believe the Anti-Kickback and Stark laws have been disastrous for medicine. Like many things, in theory it makes plenty of sense, but in practice it has led to many problems that plague physicians and subsequently patients in the end. It was passed in 1988 under President Ronald Reagan and prohibited physicians from referring patients with government-funded insurance to a laboratory they or their family had a financial interest in.

It has become even more restrictive since then, extending to the most recent amendment, which makes it illegal to receive *anything* of value for referring a patient to a facility in which the physician has an ownership, investment, or structured compensation arrangement.

The law suggests that there is an inherent conflict of interest that may adversely affect patient care. However, this restriction ignores the premise that any business has a potential conflict of interest when it comes to utilization of services or bills related to that business.

For example, it is totally legal for anyone other than a doctor to open a medical business, with or without any training, knowledge, or background in medicine and to benefit 100 percent from the care delivered on both government and commercial patients. This includes many urgent care centers and hospitals that charge exorbitant rates for simple care, laboratory evaluations, X-rays, and MRIs. But being a doctor imposes severe limitations to entrepreneurial endeavors due to potential conflicts of interest—as if only doctors can have financial conflicts in the business of medicine.

In fact, physician-owned facilities have been shown to deliver care with lower infection rates and higher patient satisfaction rates. Medicine is one of the few fields where there can be no benefit to a referring physician for sending a patient for care or surgery without facing federal indictment and criminal prosecution.

With the passage of the Affordable Care Act in 2010, President Barack Obama created task forces with a very clear objective: to identify any suggestion of improper billing (including clerical errors made by a doctor's employees) and to impose heavy penalties to include federal prosecution, turning the practice of medicine into a dangerous and scary business for doctors. The problem is that is has paved the way for unscrupulous business people to control the cost of medicine, leading to a dramatic increase in cost for patients and financial hardships for physicians.

The version of the Stark law that applies to all patients, including patients with private/commercial insurance, is called the Anti-Kickback law. Additionally, Obama also passed a law in 2010 that made it illegal for physicians to own hospitals or to expand current facilities in which they had ownership.

This enabled large hospitals with strong lobbyists to eliminate the competition provided by physician-owned hospitals. It was actually the hospital organizations that lobbied aggressively to inhibit doctors from competing with them. They argued doctors essentially couldn't be trusted, as the care delivered could be unnecessary or excessive.

A 2013 article in *American Medical News* titled "Physician-Owned Hospitals Seize Their Moment" notes that the top-performing hospital in the United States was physician-owned. Additionally, 48 of the top 100 were physician-owned.

The regulations that prohibit physicians from being entrepreneurial (i.e., having ownership in hospitals or companies that deliver healthcare services) puts that control into the hands of people more likely to care more about profit than patients, in my opinion. It ignores the fact that nearly every medical student interviewed enters medicine with a passion for helping others. We are held to higher standards than other industries even have to consider. Not only is the medical facility constantly scrutinizing the quality of care delivered by its physicians through medical staff bylaws, but those standards are upheld with peer reviews by similarly trained physicians any time there is a complication, even a complication without a breach in the standard of care. Outside of the internal facility reviews, the state medical boards are very aggressive in investigating every single allegation, frivolous or not, so much so that many physicians see their own medical boards as being unfriendly to physicians' interests.

Additionally, the vast majority of physicians are board-certified on a national level. These boards uphold high standards and often require recertification every ten years, a practice seen by many physicians as unnecessary and as a means to collect more money. All this happens in addition to the constant risk of practicing medicine in a country where frivolous lawsuits are the norm. In fact, foreign physicians are often confused at the concern American doctors express and face when practicing medicine stateside. Although like every profession, physicians have their share of unethical colleagues, the vast majority are tirelessly devoted to patient care and ethical practice. This has led many to lose their passion for our profession. It is a never-ending battle against the business owners and insurance companies who have stolen control and profitability from physicians while driving the costs of healthcare in America through the roof.

Unfortunately, doctors have neither the organization nor financial backing to battle the insurance companies or hospital lobbyists. As a result, physicians have become the pawns of big business, where money and profit are the bottom line. I am not personally aware of any physician actively encouraging their children to follow in their footsteps to become physicians. The reward of our job, which is primarily in the outcomes, is starting to become overshadowed by the worry, concern, and lack of profitability in practicing medicine. Patients are unaware of the troubles that we face and the challenges that have led to an entire country full of disenchanted, frustrated physicians. The profitability of medicine has been stolen from physicians and has been hoarded by the insurance carriers who continue to deny appropriate care in order to keep the money paid by patients for appropriate care and by hospitals who collect the vast majority of money in delivering care to patients.

In fact, a mere 10 percent of the profit of medicine is paid to physicians. The remaining 90 percent goes to the business entities within medicine. Meanwhile, doctors absorb most of the responsibility to care for and treat their patients. We must own and operate expensive medical practices with overhead increasing annually while the insurance companies continue to decrease reimbursements. This has led medicine in the wrong direction when it comes to patient care and physician satisfaction. What's alarming is that the cost of medicine continues to rise while physicians are making less, and patient care is being limited. A large percentage of physicians are closing their private practices and joining hospitals, which was probably always the plan in the first place. The long-held belief that doctors make exorbitant amounts of money has been exacerbated by federal indictments that have vilified the profession even further. The risk is beginning to outweigh the benefits for many of us. When doctors become hospital employees, the hospitals make most of the money related to patient care and pay their physicians a small percentage of what they collect.

When physicians are unable to make enough profit, they are often summarily released from the hospital. In a 2016 Medscape survey, 57 percent of physicians disagreed with workplace policy and 42 percent disagreed with their hospital over patient care. Where does this leave physicians? It seems like there's no good alternative. Patient care has become excessively expensive, which has not only led physicians to leaving their practices, but also to sometimes increasing the speed with which they deliver care. Obviously, this is an equation for disaster. As care becomes more rapid, outcomes are sure to suffer. In a profession where the vast majority of idealistic medical students entered with the idea of helping and serving others, the financial challenges—and now the criminal charges—physicians face have stolen the luster and reward of the outcomes we are working to achieve.

When one considers the fact that most physicians have the innate intelligence, drive, attention to detail, and servant-mindedness necessary to devote their lives to others, it is a shame that their offspring are now less likely to follow in their footsteps. When physicians are removed from the business side of medicine, cost escalates and care declines. Physicians are held to such high standards of care and have multiple tiers of risk when delivering care to patients, which I believe makes it far less likely they will be more unethical than those who entered the business side of medicine.

It stands to reason that this is this group, physicians, who should make decisions for patient care. They're the most at risk; they are the ones who have personal relationships and have engendered enough trust to be given the opportunity to intervene in the life and livelihood of the patient. Businessmen, on the other hand, have no real risk other than the financial and legal risk involved in patient care. They don't know the patients personally and certainly have no relationship or common trust with patients. How could they possibly care as much as physicians? Physicians can lose their licenses or lose the ability to open and operate medical facilities if things go wrong.

Many on the business side of medicine have figured out that every hospital is a lucrative real estate deal, even when the hospital fails to profit on the operations side. When their hospital fails, the owners merely close the facility and open a new one under a different name. Commonly, they open hospitals with the sole intent of making the hospital a real estate investment, flipping the hospital to a REIT then dumping the excessive cost of the operating company on the unknowing and naïve physician investors. Hospitals in which there is no physician ownership take the lion's share of the cost of the care delivered, leaving doctors to squabble over the crumbs left over from their hard work and the risk they assumed. They are protected by laws that make it illegal to help doctors operate profitable practices.

The belief that when the doctor gets paid a percentage of the profit from the work that they perform and the devices used to care for their patients automatically results in unethical behavior and overuse, which drives up cost, is a totally flawed perspective on what's happening in the operating room. Surgeons perform surgery to yield a successful result. Surgeons are the ones who should decide what should be used for their patients because they have the medical knowledge to make that determination.

They are also assuming tremendous risk in performing these procedures. Why is it seen as unethical if they benefit from a percentage or a small portion of the money being made in providing that care? Is there no risk of ethical standards being violated by anyone in this equation except doctors? Remember, doctors have scrutiny at multiple levels, including the local hospital peer review committees, the state boards, and the national boards that they're certified under—not to mention the legal risk that they face for performing unnecessary procedures. In my opinion, the most important consideration is this: Are the doctors performing unnecessary surgeries with poor outcomes in an effort to make more money? Merely making a percentage of the money that is being generated by the surgical care of a patient, does not necessarily constitute unethical behavior. It also doesn't mean that every doctor is prone to over-usage, certainly not more so than the businesspeople involved who have far less education and provide less effort in arriving at a successful outcome.

There will always be doctors who are unethical and businessmen who are unethical, but in general, doctors are ethical people who really care about the outcomes of their patients and the costs the patients absorb in receiving care. Why is it unethical for doctors to benefit financially for the work that they perform and the money that they generate? It isn't in any other industry. In the current scenario, the only people who benefit tremendously from the work being done by the doctor is the businesspeople. They make the vast majority of the money. It's not uncommon when you break down the costs paid for surgery, that the surgeon is one of the lowest paid people in the entire equation.

Even when a doctor takes 100 percent of their patients to a hospital and pays all the overhead necessary to market to patients while covering the cost to run a practice, hospitals cannot share in the marketing or general expenses of that practice. This happens while the hospitals take most of the profit in delivering patient care. Doctors also must follow their patients after surgery and continue to assume risk and responsibility in the long term over the care they delivered. This system is flawed, with doctors and patients paying the price.

Getting back to Craighead—he was definitely a strange bird. But in order to help patients that really needed spine surgery, I started to see patients at three of Craighead's clinics—San Antonio, Austin, and Corpus Christi. Contrary to what I had been led to believe, Craighead had exaggerated his patient volumes. He didn't have ninety spine patients a day per clinic! He didn't even have ten per day, for that matter. I think I saw a grand total of *three* to *four* in each of the three clinics. After three attempts to see his patients, I realized there was clearly no economic upside to this arrangement, nor was I comfortable working with Craighead, considering his eccentricities.

I informed the hospital that I felt a certain level of unease and decided to no longer see patients from his practice. My brief exposure to Craighead then ended just six months after we met when I realized that something was amiss. The exaggerated numbers of patients they supposedly had to see made me question his integrity and honesty. Coupled with his strange mannerisms, it didn't seem wise to be associated with him any further.

Meanwhile, I decided the commute to Innova was becoming a burden. Conveniently, a new hospital called Foundation was located right next to my private practice on Spurs Lane and had been empty for a year when the bariatric surgeons, for whom it was built, left. It was a beautiful facility, ideal for the kind of service I wanted to provide my patients. A friend of mine who is a bariatric surgeon and I decided to try to get that hospital up and running. We put together a group of seven surgeons to resurrect it into a multi-specialty surgical facility. (I was able to invest in the hospital by taking out a small loan from a bank.)

Everything was going well at Foundation until the chief nursing officer, who was married to an anesthesiologist on the base where I was stationed, assumed I was working during duty hours without permission. She reported me to my Air Force hospital commander and to the Pentagon. The investigation that ensued took several months and delayed me from moonlighting any further until it was complete. When the investigation concluded, it demonstrated that I had properly followed the rules (in fact, I had reported *more* hours than I worked because I always rounded up to the nearest hour.)

If only she would have asked me, I could have easily shown her the detailed logs that proved I had followed the rules. As you can imagine, I decided to leave Foundation Hospital because of how poorly this situation was handled. Thereafter, I returned to my familiar stomping grounds, Innova Hospital, where I felt confident in the integrity of the staff and their appreciation of my surgical outcomes.

Chapter Ten

Free at Last

As my time to depart the military drew near, I had many reasons to look to the future. Socially, I never really fit in at Wilford Hall. Though our department had superb residents and some great staff surgeons, the leadership had been sorely lacking ever since Dr. Parsons's departure eleven years earlier. Two other chairmen had already come and gone. As I already explained, it had become a caustic and hostile environment for me, with no love lost between me and the chairman at the time.

Typically, when personnel separate or retire from the Air Force, their department throws a big party to celebrate and to give them an appropriate send-off. But in my case, there was no party at all! This was definitely a slap in the face after fourteen years of devoted service. Typically, there is a lithograph of the hospital grounds that is signed by everyone in the department. That picture was left on my desk, totally blank, without one signature!

It was all the thanks I got for the many years of working overtime hours, assuming extra operating room days, and devoting my time to training and grooming residents to become better orthopaedic surgeons. Not to mention the countless nights of trauma call and two deployments to Iraq! Still, I was so anxious to leave that I tried not to let it bother me too much. In fact, my timing was perfect, as the morale in the department seemed to be at an all-time low.

So, on that last day, I merely walked out of the hospital with not one acknowledgment, leaving the blank lithograph where it was placed. This was certainly a shock and disappointment, considering that I had been assigned to Wilford Hall for the majority of my military career. After all, I was the chief of spine surgery and a six-year veteran professor of orthopaedic surgery—training residents, PA fellows, and medical students. Yet, in my department, there was clearly animosity against me for my success moonlighting and a personal vendetta stemming from my unwillingness to double the length of my deployment for our self-serving chairman. So, without even a simple goodbye, I was out the door. Some of the staff, residents, and PAs did arrange a going away party for me at a local restaurant to show me their gratitude and appreciation. I am grateful to them for their efforts and the opportunity to work with them over the years.

Leaving with such a bitter taste in my mouth, you can imagine my feeling when the Air Force recruiter asked me if I was ready to sign up for reserve duty to complete my twenty years of service so that I could get retirement at age sixty-five. Though I respected the Air Force as a whole, there was no way in the world I was going to sign up for even one more minute of service. Staying in reserve status would have allowed the Air Force to reactivate me, mobilize me, and deploy me anywhere the Air Force saw fit. Beaten into our heads was the motto that the "needs of the Air Force always come first." The grand total the Air Force paid for my medical school education was $69,000 since I attended a state school (University of Texas Medical School) and for that, I was required to spend fourteen years in active duty status. It was *not* a good deal financially, although there were definite benefits to my time in the military.

Though I still had tremendous respect for the military, I felt constrained and constricted by it. No longer did I want to be under the thumb of despotic leadership, controlled by a chairman who orchestrated all the unfair conditions I've described. The intrigue and backstabbing, which is present in all large institutions, but worse in my department, had worn me down.

As I look back on it, my time in the military wasn't all bad. There were times when I really loved my job. I sincerely enjoyed teaching and performing complicated surgeries. There were some amazing people who were honorable, intelligent, servant-minded patriots; some were true warriors who delivered premier care, especially when it came to trauma and wartime surgery. Then, as you've read, there were others who were far from meeting that standard, but that's human nature and it can occur in any and all fields.

As I left the Air Force, I felt grateful to the many amazing mentors who groomed me along the way and for the opportunity to help people who devoted their lives to serving our country and ensuring its safety. While we sacrificed as medical personnel when deployed, it was nothing compared to what our soldiers and combatants suffered in wartime situations. The extreme hardships and losses that they endured (and continue to bear in service to our country) deserves the utmost respect. It was an extreme honor to make personal sacrifices for them. I will be forever grateful for what they do on a daily basis for our country, as should we all.

By July 2010, I had reached my limit and was excited by the prospect of having more control over my life. No longer did I want to deploy and leave my family for extended periods of time. If I left the Air Force now, I could dictate my own schedule and would no longer have to work weekends and holidays. In short, I could actually have a normal life. It was finally time to prioritize the needs of my family, which at this time included my eight-year-old daughter, Alexa, and my five-year-old son, Caden, plus a baby due in the upcoming month. It would be a tremendous time of enjoyment for us.

On July 1, 2010, I was free and clear of my commitment to the military. My indentured servitude was over. *I was free!* And I could not have felt any happier or more relieved. I had spent fourteen years of my life dedicated to the Air Force and all that it stood for. That monumental chapter of my life was complete, allowing me to concentrate full time on building my group practice.

I was so elated about finally exiting the Air Force that we threw a massive farewell event called my "Freedom Party," inviting all our friends and close colleagues to celebrate. The party was held in our neighborhood clubhouse in San Antonio.

We decided to stay in San Antonio after my commitment to the Air Force was over. After all, my career had been built there, my father had moved the family there, and my mother and two brothers still lived there, so San Antonio was truly home. Plus, our practice had built a great reputation, so it only made sense to stay.

At this point, my philosophy of patient care was to make it as personal as possible, which was difficult when working in huge hospitals like Mayo and Wilford Hall. But like those institutions,

I wanted to continue to build a premier practice that was a one-stop shop for patients with any orthopaedic or spinal issue. But rough times were ahead.

By 2010, even before I left the Air Force, LeAnn had developed a very strong understanding of the business side of the practice. She helped to not only create The Orthopaedic & Spine Institute but also used her marketing acumen to improve our patient volume too.

So, as we added more surgeons, she had put her skills to work in the year leading up to my separation from the military. She was the architect of it all; she was in complete financial control of our affairs. She knew everything about how the practice worked and how the affiliated businesses were set up. And she did it all to the letter of the law, working with lawyers and our CPA to make sure it was compliant.

At first, our marketing had begun as a grassroots effort with LeAnn and me visiting several family practice and internal medicine clinics. On these visits, it was embarrassing and humbling to be treated like a salesperson by the front desk secretaries. Though I had never worn my physician title on my sleeve, I wasn't quite prepared for being treated like a bothersome salesman.

More often than not, I would be told that the doctors were "too busy" to see me; it was a total dismissal. Or they would spend two minutes listening to me and then scurry off and have their staff return telling me to leave a brochure or return *with lunch* in order to meet with the physicians again.

This is the problem with allowing the primary care practitioners to be the so-called "gatekeepers" of medicine. Although many of them are talented, very few of them understand who the best specialists or surgeons are. In fact, it seems that many of them don't care either way. Even when they're amazing, they are working diligently to get through the vast number of patients on their schedules, another sign that there is too heavy a push to cram patients in for a practice to succeed financially. Often, their referrals are based on their existing professional relationships instead of the training, skills, and outcomes of the specialists they refer to.

A system that gives the control over referrals to primary care physicians and incentivizes them for containing costs actually negatively impacts specialists and patients. The most effective system would include the ability of all patients, regardless of their insurance, to select whomever they choose for their care, whether it is a primary care doctor or a specialist. There should be no need to get the approval of your primary care provider to see another physician. However, many patients are required to obtain a referral from their primary care doctor, who in turn refers them to a specialist like myself. Additionally, they are encouraged to keep their patients with in-network providers. However, are the best specialists in or out of network? If a doctor is in network, they receive reduced rates from the insurance companies with the promise of getting more patients, who never come. The in-network system is a huge scam.

The insurance carriers' promise of additional patient volume never came to fruition for specialists and created the idea that primary care physicians should be the gatekeepers of medicine, determining whether a patient should be sent for specialty care. As the insurance carriers captured more physicians in their network by diverting patients only to these in-network doctors, more physicians began to join the networks. Eventually, it became almost impossible to have any patient volume if a physician stayed out of network to avoid the drastic cuts in their reimbursements. But "incentives" for patients to go to in-network doctors and financial penalties for going out of network forced most patients to stay in their network of physicians. This tactic proved effective for the insurance carriers. Now with control of the patients and network rates, they had us where they wanted us, in the palm of their hands. They could decrease our reimbursements at will, and they have. The carriers are happy to charge for out-of-network insurance coverage but pull out all the stops, essentially coaxing and threatening patients with huge financial penalties for going out of network. Everything's under the table, secret, and skewed toward financial benefit to the insurance companies. Insurance companies act as if the money paid to them by patients is theirs to control, instead of the patients' investment in their health.

So, what they'll do is pay a crummy contracted rate to in-network doctors and facilities. And even then, my clinic has been forced on occasion to sue multiple insurance companies to collect the money that should've come to us in the first place, based on our contracted rates, splitting the money ultimately collected with a collection lawyer, who typically takes 50 percent.

On what basis do they deny such claims? *They make it up.* You didn't dot an i; you forgot to put a dash between your social security number; the pre-authorizations weren't properly filed. And even when they are approved, they have a disclaimer on all pre-authorizations that state that *authorization is not a guarantee of payment*! Because they have access to your bank account, they can literally go into it and claw back the money they've paid you without your approval. And you better believe, they actually do that! How in the world does that happen? It's like a plumber charging me $3,000 to fix my pipes. I agree to the fee but after the work is complete, I only pay them ten dollars because I changed my mind.

Meanwhile, from the vantage point of the patient, the insurance companies basically control them as well. If they go out of network because they found a better doctor, they're going to be penalized and pay more money. It is not uncommon to get denials for care, for medicine, or for procedures. The only winner in this system is the insurance company.

Because primary care doctors are the "gatekeepers," they often dictate when and where patients go for specialty care. This places an additional financial burden on specialists to perform direct marketing to patients with PPO insurance, who don't require referrals for specialty care, in order to make up for lost HMO referrals, an additional financial burden to private practice.

LeAnn's frustration with grassroots marketing prompted a new strategy. She decided to take the marketing directly *to* the patients instead of begging for HMO and government referrals from primary care doctors. This was an unorthodox strategy for the San Antonio market that had only been used by slick plastic surgeons and ambulance-chasing lawyers. Traditionally, any physician marketing themselves commercially had been frowned upon; it was viewed as unprofessional. But we were outside-the-box thinkers and refused to be held hostage by primary care doctors and pain specialists with established referral patterns to other doctors based on friendships (and crony lunches). We felt then, and still believe today, that referrals must be based on the *quality* of your work and the integrity of your practice.

Patients deserved real options based on their own research, not their doctors' relationships. In our view, marketing directly to patients would allow them to figure out who we were and what we stood for. If done correctly, it would give them a glimpse into our specific area of expertise and our successful surgical outcomes, a record that separated us from the pack. LeAnn believed that a marketing plan that highlighted my training and experience would be very helpful in improving my presence in the city. And as always, she was correct.

To market me and the practice, she initiated a campaign, spending money for billboards, radio spots, and TV segments. It was highly effective; and my volume of patients climbed rapidly from having one evening clinic per week to a busy, five-day-a-week clinical practice.

Over the preceding six years, from 2004 to 2010, word of mouth had already begun to spread about my surgical outcomes. But now, with more patient traffic produced by the ads, direct referrals began to arrive even faster. I was forced to hire more mid-level providers to coordinate conservative care prior to considering surgery.

As the practice grew rapidly, we began fielding requests from multiple other doctors to join us. Pain specialists, spine surgeons, adult and pediatric orthopaedic surgeons, neurologists, vascular surgeons, dermatologists, plastic surgeons, and three family practice doctors *all* requested to join me after seeing the success and rapid growth of my practice.

LeAnn and I felt that creating this kind of multi-specialty practice would enable us to keep our care in-house, which would lead to more reliable patient outcomes. It allowed us to control the type of care our patients received and from whom. Having all our services in-house unfortunately created political turmoil in our community, because I was no longer referring to *other* practices, such as pain management and physical therapy. Those practitioners now saw me as competition. So instead of referring to me, they would bash me in order to convince their patients to see doctors they had relationships with.

My approach to medicine was quite different than theirs because it was not based on an economic motive. Whereas I wanted to cure a patient's condition and eliminate the need for a specialist (including me), some pain doctors and chiropractors wanted to hold on to their patients and turn them into a perpetual revenue stream. I have always held to the philosophy that it's better to be busy from word-of-mouth marketing that results from great outcomes than from working fast, cutting corners, and increasing revenue from an assembly line–style practice. I spend a lot of time with my patients, both to understand their condition and to get to know them as people. The revenue may be lower with that approach, but your reward will be far greater in the end. If you serve a higher purpose, the benefit is eternal. I think it's easy to fall into the trap of flying through surgery and clinic to make more money, or to get home at a certain hour, but those patients are putting their trust and lives in our hands. We owe them every ounce of effort we have to improve their condition.

Connecting to patients and empathizing with their condition cannot happen in a fifteen-minute visit. It is also very important to educate patients about their conditions and the options to treat them and the restrictions they should follow to ensure an optimal result. Despite the ever-decreasing reimbursement, physicians must focus on treating their patients like they would their own families or how they'd expect to be treated if they were the patient. That philosophy has helped me deliver the best for every person I treat. No surgeon or physician is perfect, and we all have cases that could have gone better. We all have complications. They say, "You cut, you cry." It means that we will all have outcomes that we wish were better, but with this approach and good training, they should be rare.

In 2011, a year after my return to Innova, I heard that Andrew Hillman and the owner of Innova, Bob Helms, had decided to partner up to create a Texas-wide hospital system that would match the success they were experiencing at Innova in San Antonio. The plan was to create the so-called Victory Hospital Group, an eight-hospital system in Dallas, Ft. Worth, Houston, and San Antonio.

To me, this rapid expansion plan seemed a bit aggressive and risky. Yet, they forged ahead and even decided to build a brand-new hospital in San Antonio too, replacing the one I was accustomed to. However, there were early signs that Innova was going to have financial struggles doing all this. There were delays in reimbursements and denials in payment from the insurance companies to Innova because of their out-of-network status. Although insurance carriers have options for out-of-network coverage, which costs patients and their employers quite a bit more than in-network-only plans, they try really hard to prevent their clients from using that benefit. Out of network means that the facility or physician seeing or treating the patient has not agreed to fee reductions, therefore the cost is higher. Insurance carriers try to discourage patients by making them responsible for 50 percent of the cost, whereas with an in-network provider the patient responsibility is, for example, 20 percent. Meanwhile, the insurance carrier is charging a higher premium for that benefit. So it stands to reason that they can increase their profit margins if they take the higher monthly premiums for the benefit, but patients never use their out-of-network coverage. When that fails to work and patients seek out-of-network care regardless (often for a facility or physician who is worth the extra cost), the insurance carrier scares the patients about how expensive it will be with their 50 percent responsibility. They then pay the facility or physician extremely slowly, and sometimes not at all.

This was the case with Innova. Several insurance carriers owed the hospital tens of millions of dollars for care that was already pre-authorized and delivered and didn't seem motivated to pay. They basically decided they wouldn't pay. What could this little hospital do about it? They had enough money to fight in court for as long as necessary and could easily outspend a physician group or small hospital like Innova. Obviously, this lost revenue after the expense necessary to perform surgeries and care for patients was a huge financial blow to the hospital.

Now that Andrew was involved in the San Antonio hospital, we spoke often about how to help make the hospital more successful. He talked about his many business ventures and the capital he had to build on that empire. In discussions with Andrew, the idea about my desire to create my own implant line came up. I explained to him that I felt frustrated that Allure was taking so long to produce the implants we had been working on in research development. It was at this point that Andrew started discussing his interest in getting into the surgical implant business. Andrew suggested that he could partner with Allure to expedite the process because he had the influence to make it happen on a larger scale, or so he said.

This alliance would also allow us to obtain licensing agreements with the long-term goal of getting my designs to market. It sounded like a good plan to me. I would serve as a consultant and chief medical officer to a new implant company, which was now named Total Surgical Management; Allure would be our initial supplier. At Total Surgical, my role was slightly more involved, in that I would provide medical insight and recommendations as well as design ideas for the future.

Prior to 2011, one of Andrew's many businesses also included a pharmacy in the University of Texas Southwestern medical office building, one that provided prescription drugs for workers' compensation patients. This traditional pharmacy concept would later be expanded to include a "compounding" pharmacy for pain creams, which was a relatively new therapeutic modality at the time. Compounding pharmacies had developed a novel way to incorporate prescription pain medications into creams that could be applied topically. The theory and benefit of these preparations was that they eliminated the potential side effects of taking narcotics, steroids, anti-inflammatory medications, muscle relaxants, and nerve pain medications in pill form.

The idea of using these creams in my practice had been introduced to me by both my brother Bryan (always on the lookout for innovations in medicine) and by one of my nurse practitioners, Sharon, who had benefited greatly from the creams as a patient herself.

I admit that I was somewhat skeptical of these compounded products until I witnessed firsthand how effective they actually were. Patient after patient reported significant improvement in pain from the creams without sedation, constipation, or nausea associated with the pill forms of the medications. It was genius really.

The safety of this form of pain relief was intriguing to me because narcotic medications and all their side effects create a litany of woes for both surgeons and patients. In my experience, patients undergoing surgery who had taken narcotics prior to surgery were always the most miserable.

Their postoperative pain relief was almost impossible to achieve because they had built up a tolerance to the pain medications. Therefore, compounded pain creams would theoretically allow us to treat preoperative and postoperative pain without heavy narcotics, thus avoiding addiction, tolerance, and poor post-surgery pain relief. To me, this was especially important, as the opioid addiction rate in America was skyrocketing at the time, with more than 70,000 overdose deaths in America annually.

At this point, when Bryan introduced the idea of compounding creams to Andrew, he loved the idea and created an entire team to implement this new business model into his portfolio, which included sixty-seven businesses, according to his exaggerated accounting. On top of using the compounding creams in our practice, we also consulted with a pain management specialist and established protocols for toxicology testing in our clinic.

In addition to the risk of doing surgery on patients with narcotic medications on board, doctors also constantly worry about non-prescription medications or medications that patients fail to admit they're taking when we're performing surgery on them. There have been multiple instances of patients having a stroke or heart attack because they were on illicit drugs that no one was aware of. To avoid these types of complications intraoperatively, along with avoiding other complications related to prescribing medications when someone is taking illicit drugs, toxicology screening became standard. In fact, multiple doctors in Texas had been sanctioned in recent years after adverse events in their patients resulted from narcotic overdosing and interactions. It became a Texas law and the Texas Medical Board made it mandatory to perform toxicology screening and to create pain contracts between doctors and patients.

This was even more incentive to ensure that it was very clear what patients were taking prior to and after surgery. So, in an effort to improve patient safety, we implemented toxicology screening into our practice as well. In my view, housing the screening right inside the practice was the best way to identify patients taking illicit drugs, ensuring that patients could not evade testing and move ahead with their surgeries anyway. It was all about patient safety. Putting these protocols in place required quite a bit of work, creating policies and protocols in the clinic that had not been implemented previously.

With this in mind, LeAnn envisioned a marketing company that would teach doctors how to implement toxicology testing in their clinics. Many of the toxicology testing companies began to allow doctors to become investors in their companies. But this was a tricky scenario because once a doctor invested, they had to make sure they didn't violate any of the Anti-Kickback or Stark regulations related to patient referrals.

In order to understand the compliance issues related to these physician investments in any medical company, LeAnn consulted with both our longtime personal healthcare attorney and Andrew's primary attorney, Nick Oberheiden. Understanding how to be entrepreneurial while maintaining compliance with the Anti-Kickback laws was vital. None of us wanted to bend, let alone break, the law. Every process and protocol we implemented was sent to both attorneys to review and approve. I never relied solely on the attorney assigned to a business for my own legal advice. LeAnn and I knew how important it was to have an independent attorney represent our personal interests, just in case the attorney representing a business had a hidden agenda. So our healthcare attorney was always a vital part of our plan to stay compliant. This caution saved our hides, as you will see.

Chapter Eleven

"Cutter"

With our business interests in the hospital, investments in Andrew's lab, and the implant company intermingled with Andrew's managerial hand, it wasn't always easy, to say the least. He was a very dominating, disrespectful, aggressive kind of manager.

At one point, LeAnn had tried to help several of our friends by having them work for Andrew's companies, but being an employee in one of his companies was not a pleasant experience according to several of them. We were told more than once that he was a despot, and that he was crude and frequently inappropriate. His employees complained that he drove his employees' salaries down while driving up his business profits and the salaries of his executive staff.

Eventually, multiple friends of ours who joined Andrew to try to build his implant company in the beginning left disgruntled and frustrated. This particularly upset us because, in our lives as

Christians, relationships mean far more than profits. Yet, we could not control the uncontrollable Andrew.

A fallout with Andrew was inevitable. We weren't equally yoked as people nor as business partners, and I would eventually see through his continuous lies and manipulations. In the fall of 2013, Andrew introduced to us yet another one of his enterprises, a wellness and weight-loss company called Health Crave based in Dallas. He suggested that we could introduce Health Crave into our practice to assist patients in losing weight in advance of surgery. I knew a weight-loss program would be highly beneficial, because a lot of patients who are overweight experience increased joint and back pain and face much higher complication rates in surgery.

LeAnn envisioned expanding the Health Crave brand and creating an entire wellness division within our practice, incorporating a non-surgical component that could later expand into other physicians' practices as well. The concept was that we could offer other physicians a plan for how to incorporate multiple lines of services like toxicology, pharmacy, hormone therapy, and weight loss, etc., into their practices to take care of the "whole patient" through preventative medicine.

In the fall of 2013, LeAnn decided to take this project on herself with the approval of Andrew and his Health Crave partners. We were the flagship office for this new plan to vertically integrate healthcare. LeAnn worked tirelessly on this project and hired and trained multiple marketing representatives to help her. She also subcontracted multiple third-party marketing firms to expand her bandwidth throughout central and south Texas.

Her focus was on branding and expanding the Health Crave concept through direct marketing to the public via billboards, radio and television ads, networking events, and good old-fashioned door-to-door marketing. Although effective, the venture proved to be extremely expensive, far exceeding the payments received by LeAnn for her services.

Concurrently, the compounding pharmacy and toxicology screening industry took off like wildfire, not only with Andrew's companies, but also with multiple other companies around the state and across the nation. A protocol that was initially built as a safety mechanism for both patients and physicians became very lucrative for the businesspeople involved.

Most of the toxicology labs were out of network, which led to exorbitant fees, infuriating the insurance carriers and patients alike. On the business side, the dollar figures being billed to the insurance companies were astronomical. Doctors had no say in what these pharmacies or labs billed, but they were prescribing the compounds and testing with increased frequency, assuming this newfound strategy would promote patient safety.

Andrew began allowing physicians to invest in his toxicology labs, where no government patients were being tested. However, I would later discover that he also set up other labs that were performing toxicology screening on government patients. He hired marketers from all over the state and created a new company with no physician partners that housed all his toxicology labs and compounding companies; it was called NextHealth. It became his most lucrative business by far, so much so, that he began to neglect all his other enterprises, including the implant company we had worked so hard to create. His interest in branding Health Crave also waned as he was quickly on to bigger and better projects with many new partners we had never met and who were increasingly disrespectful to us and dismissive of our business interests in south Texas.

In 2014, just as my practice looked like it was reaching the pinnacle of success, with twenty-two medical providers and a hundred-plus staff, I had one of the biggest scares of my life. Julia Eller, the owner of Allure, (the implant company I had been doing consulting work for) was federally indicted along with a nationally recognized Army spine surgeon, Lieutenant Colonel Rick Rooney. Rooney pled guilty for what the government charged was a $7.3 million healthcare fraud scheme. The implications for me were that, since I was previously affiliated with Allure in my design efforts/consulting agreement, I would now be heavily scrutinized. When these things happen, the government casts a wide net to investigate all affiliated entities to identify any other violations of the law. Even if you are innocent, they will look closely at your contracts and arrangements to verify it.

The sixty-five-count indictment alleged that, over a period of eight years (2002–2010), Allure paid Rooney, his wife (who was also a doctor), and his father-in-law kickbacks for the use of Allure's products on Rooney's military patients. Moreover, it was alleged that Rooney hid his financial interest in Julia's medical device company. He had other problems as well: this happened while he was active duty, and he had not been granted commander approval to moonlight (i.e., to receive money outside his military salary). So even if he had a legitimate arrangement with Allure, it would have been a problem with the military.

While Julia dodged prison time and only served probation, Rooney was tried and ultimately sentenced to a nearly three-year jail term. Although I didn't know Rooney well, he had a great reputation as a talented surgeon with outstanding outcomes and training. Word has it that he pled because the federal attorney threatened to go after his wife and father-in-law, but he was innocent of the charges.

Yes, he was convicted of being paid by Allure and Altiva (another implant company) in exchange for using their devices in his surgeries, but if this kind of thing happened in any other profession, such an arrangement would create no legal repercussions.

I was learning that physicians were in a special kind of jeopardy regarding anything financial or entrepreneurial. In other words, according to the U.S. government, doctors are supposed to be purely practitioners, *not* entrepreneurs. Any attempt to be entrepreneurial is met with skepticism, even amongst other physicians. We have become brainwashed to think making a profit is unethical. Corporate America uses that sentiment to push doctors and nurses to the brink physically trying to do what's right for their patients, even when they're struggling financially and physically to do so. They bank on that conscientiousness then shame and pursue doctors who try to invest in medical business ventures. But since doctors care the most about their patients, and have multiple layers of liability, whether it be medical malpractice or ethics issues, why *shouldn't* they be able to benefit from the business side of medicine? And, why were they being punished more harshly than the businesspeople who dragged them into the agreement that was considered illegal in the first place? The double standard is concerning. Why shouldn't the business owner, who created the agreement, be held to a *higher* standard than the person who was baited into the situation to begin with? Doctors are being indicted, convicted, and going to federal prison. They lose their license to practice medicine in the process. So even when they've paid their time, they get out of jail stripped of their ability to practice medicine while the businesspeople continue to run businesses in the medical field without restrictions.

In 2007, five of the largest implant manufacturers of orthopaedic and spinal implants—Zimmer, Stryker, Smith+Nephew, Biomet, and DePuy—were charged with providing kickbacks to doctors for using their products. All except Stryker paid a hefty fine, totaling $311 million, but none of the administrators did jail time. Doctors reportedly were paid tens to hundreds of thousands of dollars per year by these companies. The U.S. attorney who prosecuted the case noted that "doctors made decisions based on how much money they could make," not on the best interests of their patients. Although that comment may have been accurate for some, I am confident the vast majority of these physicians would have used the same products regardless. Most surgeons are loyal to a company's products because they trained with those products in their residencies or fellowships, or found that the products were reliable and user-friendly. Many of them are already using a specific company's implants before ever being offered consulting arrangements.

In June of 2021, *Fortune* published an article entitled "The Spinal Tap: Device makers have funneled billions to orthopedic surgeons who use their products." The author laments how, over the course of six years between 2013 and 2019, a "torrent of cash and other compensation [totaling $3.1 billion] flows" to surgeons, according to a KHN analysis. Although that number sounds extreme, it is for six years and for every single surgeon performing design work and even creating novel implants for orthopaedic and spine surgery. The same article goes on to say that treatment for back pain and worn-out joints tops $20 billion annually. It also notes that orthopedic and neurosurgeons collected more than $500 million dollars for consulting between 2013 and 2020. So the very surgeons creating and improving surgical implants make a small fraction of the profits from these implants for their efforts. Why is there a problem with that? To be clear—I'm not referring to illegal kickbacks. I'm referring to legitimate design and intellectual property arrangements that lead to improved care and the evolution of surgery. To assume the small payments of tens to hundreds of thousands of dollars in an entire year are extreme is to ignore the fact that equipment companies can make that in **one case** with a surgeon. The financial benefit is primarily theirs and the hospital's, with surgeons bringing in a small fraction of the money paid, even when they have consulting agreements. The assumption that a doctor's involvement in a business automatically results in unethical behavior is a totally flawed view of reality. Surgeons, specifically, have tremendous incentive to do precisely what their patients need. They assume tremendous risk in performing these surgeries. When a physician performs surgeries with poor outcomes, when patients are being injured in surgery, it's usually their physician colleagues who report them. We definitely hold each other accountable more than most other professions. We are all called to "do no harm," which is the minimum standard; no physician likes seeing another physician hurt patients. Christopher Duntsch, aka "Dr. Death," for example, was turned in to the Texas Medical Board by fellow physicians for his gross negligence and malpractice, not the hospital staff nor administrators. We police each other very well. Doctors are even hypercritical of each other.

I believe the key issue to consider is this: Are the doctors performing unnecessary procedures or surgeries with poor outcomes in an effort to make more money? Merely making a percentage of the money generated in the care of a patient does not necessarily constitute unethical behavior. It also doesn't mean that every doctor is prone to over-usage, but doctors are human so they aren't all ethical. They should be watched for unethical patterns and bad outcomes. However, to hold them to a standard that no one else is held to either inside or outside their industry is frankly inhibiting cost containment and quality care. Surgeons and physicians in general care about their patients, even the costs they absorb to receive care. I believe we would fight to contain cost, within reason, out of concern for our patients. As it stands, often the surgeon is the lowest paid entity represented in the operating room. As I've stated previously, every business entity in the room—the hospital, the equipment companies, even their vendors, the anesthesiologists, even—make more money than the person doing the surgery. That doesn't even make sense. That being said, I believe the law should always be adhered to, regardless of how illogical it may be. It's just not worth the risk or penalty one faces when the government comes after you.

But, why is this the law? Everyone stands to make money in the business of medicine. If doctors do most of the work, why are they the smallest piece of the pie? Why can't they partake in the financial reward that the businesspeople enjoy while following strict guidelines for ethical practice? Maybe a better solution is to have transparency into the surgeries performed and the cost assumed when a doctor is involved in the hospital or implant company. It's definitely possible to ensure surgeons aren't over-utilizing services by comparing to past performance and volumes prior to entering these agreements or to set up a standard by which they must comply to ensure ethical practice.

Not surprisingly, of course, the press has a field day with stories of "fraud," "kickbacks," and "greedy doctors." It certainly makes for a sexy headline, even more so than stories about unethical businessmen. Though my affiliation and design services were with the same company (Allure) that was involved in the indictment with Rooney, my contract was quite different.

First, I *had* been given commander approval to moonlight. Second, I had an intellectual property agreement with Allure that was drawn up by my certified healthcare attorney. Third, I did not use the products I was designing on military or government patients. Fourth, as recommended by my attorney, I charged fair market value for the design and consulting work I did, following every one of his recommendations to a tee (like the typical rule follower that I am!). Fifth, I had extensive documentation to back all this up, including invoices that were meticulously organized, thanks to LeAnn. Bottom line, my arrangement with Allure was totally legal.

Unfortunately, after this story hit the headlines, because I was also affiliated with Allure, the federal attorney in charge of the case sent a grand jury subpoena for *my* records, including detailed invoices with drawings, timelines, technique guides, dated email correspondence, and research I had conducted.

For months, I was in a panic. One of the attorneys who represented me spoke ominously about my likelihood of being indicted so I would hire him to represent me. I ended up engaging him plus another federal healthcare attorney to defend me for a whopping $65,000—an amount I did not have—to prove that I had not violated the law. An FBI agent even posed as a patient in my clinic and then questioned several people who knew me to determine if I was ethical.

In the end, my intellectual property agreement with Allure was deemed legally compliant when all my documentation verified my work effort. I proved I earned the little bit of money I was paid and had never received a kickback, so the issue was dropped. Fortunately, I had set up my consulting agreement correctly. I had detailed invoices based on industry-standard hourly payments for a spine surgeon, detailed drawings, technique guides, articles and information I had researched, and an intellectual property agreement drawn up by my healthcare attorney that all parties complied with. But boy, was that a scary experience! LeAnn and I were obviously alarmed by the turn of all these events.

As a spine surgeon, from day one, multiple vendors and businessmen had approached me about investing in their companies, doing medical research and consulting, or getting involved in the design of medical equipment and the development of intellectual property. There were also options offered for a physician-owned implant distributorship. I never felt comfortable with these offers because it didn't appear that any of those companies were looking for novel ideas but were merely hoping to rope the surgeons into using their implants.

As I observed from the example of other ambitious physicians in the news, even an innocent attempt to be entrepreneurial could lead to indictments, convictions, and at a minimum, tarnished reputations. Businessmen were preying on surgeons, banking on their lack of understanding of the healthcare regulations, leading physicians to violating the law without even knowing it.

This predatory approach to surgeons spanned the spectrum from hospital owners and marketing and implant companies to toxicology labs, pharmacies, and even to other doctors and physicians. I had run into innumerable people claiming they could help me grow my patient volume, increase my revenue, and even make me a millionaire. These vultures typically seek out doctors, particularly surgeons, as easy prey. We obviously have little training in business and even less in the laws that determine ethical business practices. If a surgeon fails to learn these rules of engagement on their own or fails to seek the advice of an ethical healthcare attorney (and follow it), they can easily fall victim to a host of different money-making schemes that get them into hot water. In extreme cases, such missteps may even lead to the physician losing their license or ending up in prison.

I had the misfortune to make the acquaintance of a businessman/chiropractor and former part owner of Innova Hospital. He was constantly trying to figure out how to personally capitalize on my business. When I began doing surgeries at Innova, he offered me a 25 percent ownership in the profits of an implant company he was affiliated with. I had no interest in that type of arrangement and politely declined.

Later, he scheduled a meeting with me and LeAnn, having figured out she had a lot to do with the business side of our practice. In that meeting, I realized why I never liked him. He would refer to all surgeons as "cutters," which was to me a very derogatory term. This guy would go out and recruit older surgeons who were in the twilight of their careers, well into their late sixties or seventies, to perform surgeries with little to no workup or an established doctor/patient relationship. Nearly all of the surgeries were performed on Department of Labor employees with work-related injuries.

The degrading way he talked about surgeons really irked me, as if we were there just to cut, like butchers, with no compassion, integrity, or positive purpose other than making money, ignoring the amount of their clinical knowledge and skill, along with the risk a surgeon takes, when caring for a patient. But my purpose was far greater than money, and far higher than the assembly line mentality of lining people up to be "cut open." The term cutters relegated us to mindless butchers; and I resented the reference.

After all, it took me until I was thirty-two years old to complete all my medical and surgical education. The training was intense, challenging, and laborious. We learned the intricacies of the human body like no other profession. Our purpose was to heal, to correct a malady, to eliminate a life-altering problem when no other option could provide a solution. It's why I became a surgeon in the first place. Our mission was to intervene with a definitive outcome. So his derogatory attitude toward doctors left me disgusted. LeAnn and I left that meeting realizing that a lot of businessmen like this bozo viewed surgeons as their pawns and patients as a means to a financial end. I vowed to never do anything with that guy. He was a despicable human in my eyes.

This is why physicians must be involved on the business side of medicine. Otherwise, people with no standards, no risk, and no repercussions make decisions based solely on profits, without consideration for what it takes to be a doctor or a surgeon or even the struggles of being a patient. In order to initiate change, physicians are going to have to eventually bond together to advocate for themselves and patients against this tyrannical system, which turns us into pawns for every scoundrel on the business side of the equation. Few people really understand what it takes, not just the number of years we train, but what sacrifices we make to have the privilege of being physicians. If they had it their way, we would be mindless technicians who they could control both physically and financially—which is already happening.

I just wanted to innovate and improve patient care and safety and have a line of implants I could proudly call my own, just as some of my mentors had done at Mayo. However, as I say, the idea of massive wealth had never entered my mind, nor did it motivate me. It wasn't about to start now. If money was my focus in becoming a physician, I never would have entered the military in the first place.

But now I asked myself, *What kind of business have I gotten into?* This was not at all what I had envisioned. Here I was attempting to create an implant line of my own that would be hugely beneficial to my patients, and what was happening? Doctors who devoted their lives to helping others were being federally indicted, convicted, and sent to jail for *consulting* agreements. And as you'll see, things would only get worse.

Chapter Twelve

To Lease or Not to Lease

Outside of my desire to innovate, my primary focus, of course, was taking care of patients. From the time we created The Orthopaedic & Spine Institute in 2005 to its peak in 2013, the practice grew exponentially, from just me and my trusted nurse practitioner, Eloy, to a total of twenty-two providers!

By 2013, there were three family practice doctors, a vascular surgeon, a neurologist, a dermatologist, a plastic surgeon, three pain doctors, two pediatric orthopaedic surgeons, two general orthopaedic surgeons (including a hand surgeon), and three spine surgeons, including me. On top of that, when you added in all the PAs, nurse practitioners, and administrative support, we had a total staff of 105!

To provide adequate office space and enough exam rooms, we kept absorbing adjacent space. The practice was forced to grow from its original footprint of 3,500 square feet in 2007 to a whopping 20,000 square feet by 2013. Our overhead was fearsome—the rent was now $60,000 per month, plus an additional $300,000 monthly to cover operating costs. In retrospect, this rapid expansion was certainly an unwise business decision considering the "team" I had assembled; and it eventually would lead to a total collapse of our practice.

One would think this massive group of providers and staff would be able to generate enough money to pay the overhead, but there are many factors in play here that led to a total collapse of our practice. One of the primary issues is the insurance company's stranglehold on reimbursements and denials of care, delay in payments, and outright control of physicians' incomes. The current system allows the insurance carriers to dictate what services are worth, what a doctor should be paid, and the sole discretion of whether or not to pay even after the care has been provided. The current system is a huge farce. To pull off this scam, insurance companies get around the Corporate Practice of Medicine Doctrine by hiring physicians to ration and deny care. This act was intended to prevent corporations, businesses, or outside entities from hindering a physician from delivering care they deemed appropriate for their patients. It was intended to prevent corporations from interfering with patient care for the sole purpose of profit. It is violated every single day through the "peer-to-peer" review process implemented by insurance carriers. They have identified a loophole that needs to be closed immediately, as it violates the intent of this act and inhibits physicians from taking adequate care of their patients.

Here's how they do it: The carriers hire doctors, many of whom are retired, to deny tests, treatment, and even surgeries requested by the treating physician. Because it's a physician denying the care, the insurance carriers have been able to get around the notion that they are practicing medicine. However, these denials typically begin with a nurse. Yes, a nurse denies doctors' requests for treatment. When that happens, if the doctor requests an appeal or reconsideration, the insurance company may (I emphasize *may*) allow a peer-to-peer discussion. These doctors are rarely peers. Oftentimes, the peer-to-peer is performed with a "medical director," usually an internal medicine doctor with zero experience in surgery. They couldn't even sew up a wound in most cases, let alone weigh in on complex surgical indications and treatments. Sometimes it's a retired doctor in a similar specialty, but often it's not. It's an ob-gyn, pediatrician, or general surgeon weighing in on the care requested from a spine specialist, for example.

I have performed many peer-to-peer reviews with people who had no clue about the surgery or treatment they were denying. They had no background or experience and certainly no expertise in the field they were denying or rationing care in. They were making medical decisions for patient care when they didn't even have the credentials or privileges to perform the treatments they were denying. Often these doctors are from another state. They don't even have a license to practice in the state where their decisions are controlling care. Even when these peer-to-peer doctors are of the same specialty, it's irrelevant what they think. They have a hidden agenda to deny care. It's also common for specialists to disagree on the best treatment. That's why we have to train for so long. It's incumbent upon the patient to make wise decisions about who they're seeing, so they go to doctors with good training and a reputation for good outcomes. But peer-to-peer doctors were hired specifically with the goal of denying care and increasing profits. If the insurance carrier wanted what was best for the patient, they would approve the care without any fuss, considering the doctor requesting treatment had the appropriate credentials to render the care requested.

Lord knows the peer-to-peer doctors don't have appropriate credentials. Literally *none* of them have ever spoken with or examined the patients they are preventing from having much-needed medical intervention or surgery. Moreover, there are no legal repercussions or financial risks to their denials. While the patients suffer from delayed treatment, these peer-to-peer doctors walk off with their couple of hundred dollars for each review. The insurance companies get their way—they keep more of the patients' money. In fact, the more these peer-to-peer doctors deny, the more often they are likely to be hired. I faced that scenario earlier in my career, as I described, when my frequent approvals were met with requests by the insurance carriers to stop using me as a reviewer.

And what's even more insane is that even when authorization is granted, the insurance carrier attaches a disclaimer to the approval that says, "Pre-authorization is not a guarantee of payment." And to prove that, there have been many instances in which I performed a surgery, the carrier enlisted a sell-out doctor to deny the treatment retrospectively, and then they took the money out of our corporate bank account without our approval or knowledge beforehand! Not only did they deny my payment after surgery, but they stiffed everyone involved in that surgery too: the hospital, the anesthesiologist, the neuromonitoring company, the vascular surgeon, the first assistant, the implant company, the durable medical equipment company—everyone. The care was approved. It was provided. Risk and cost to provide that surgery in addition to the effort necessary to perform a surgery were assumed without getting paid. That doesn't happen in any other industry. Why isn't that a crime?!

We thought that expanding our clinic would enable us to treat a greater number of patients more effectively. Many of the doctors that we had entrusted our businesses to failed to deliver. For example, there were only four doctors in our practice, including me, who actually generated more revenue than their personal overhead. The others, like the three family practitioners, had unreasonably high demands but low output, and they became a complete drain on the practice. The family practice doctors, for example, generated no profit for the practice but had demanded their own suite of offices with nine exam rooms requiring me to acquire a 6,700-square-foot space just for them! I tried to offset the cost of the additional space we acquired by purchasing an MRI machine to generate additional revenue. Afterall, we ordered more than 100 MRIs as a group per month.

The family practice doctors essentially worked part time. One of them had to leave by 3:00 p.m. each day and worked three days per week but still demanded three exam rooms to accommodate her patients. The other two complained incessantly about any and everything. It was no wonder their practice was failing before they joined mine. And now they were all dragging us down with them.

All these bad business decisions combined with poor insurance reimbursement and staff who didn't pull their weight was leading toward our financial disaster. Additionally, our office manager, who had done a great job for the years preceding, was frankly overwhelmed, unable to keep up administratively with our rapid expansion. Not only that, but multiple staff members reported that they couldn't find her on the premises. She hired high school friends, whom she failed to supervise to the extent that they felt free to sit around and gossip, take lunch without clocking out, have their friends clock them in at 8:00 a.m., and show up one to two hours late. Many of the staff failed to bill, or to verify insurance coverage. When the insurance companies played their typical tricks by refusing to pay for the care we provided, the billing department staff neglected to resubmit claims for payment.

Despite the lack of revenue the doctors were generating, they didn't seem to care or understand that they had a responsibility for the part of their individual overhead. They viewed their guaranteed paycheck as a foregone conclusion, as they demanded high-dollar equipment and luxurious clinic space. When I look back on it, I can see all the cracks in the wall, so to speak.

In an effort to stop the bleeding, we hired a healthcare compliance expert and auditor, Linda D'Spain, to evaluate the practice. We hoped her skills would allow us to improve efficiency while also ensuring that proper protocols were in place for continued compliance. Our previous office manager was highly insulted by the idea of having someone audit *her* work, but the practice was truly a mess.

The auditor confirmed the obvious—that we had too many staff, including the physicians, who were not carrying their weight. She noted that it was highly irregular that these in-house physicians would not be required to cover their own personal overhead. I was told that the contract we had for the physicians was not stringent enough and that the agreements needed to be renegotiated to save the practice.

She recommended an industry-standard management fee above the individual cost to practice, giving each physician an opportunity to determine the number of staff they needed to support their practice. Preceding this audit, we started having regular meetings to discuss efficiency and cross-pollination by the physicians within the practice in order to optimize our success, but it fell mainly on deaf ears.

Indeed, no matter what I said or recommended, no physician in my group practice changed their work effort or ethic. They took for granted the extensive and expensive marketing we had undertaken to boost volume and recognition for all our specialists. At one point, we had thirteen billboards, a recurring TV commercial shown during the Spurs games, multiple radio ads, plus paid-for television appearances for our physicians. We were also optimizing Google AdWords for each specialty and each physician individually.

How did we fund all these costs? We did it primarily by deferring both my income in the clinic and using profit distributions from the hospital (at least for the one year it was profitable) to pay the clinic's overhead. Despite absorbing all these costs, it just wasn't enough. And as the practice began to flounder, we were eventually unable to cover our overhead at all; we were even forced to cash out our kids' college savings plans.

In the fall of 2015, as a last-ditch effort, our auditor discussed with our physicians a new contract that would obligate them to earn their keep and pay for their share of our expenses, but instead they stampeded out the door!

Nearly every one of them decided to leave us. Only the three physicians closest to me, my Bible-study *Christian* brothers, decided to stay, or so they led me to believe. Unfortunately, during this tumultuous period, I had just signed a six-year extension on my clinic lease, and as the sole owner of the practice, I was the only one responsible for *all* financial costs. So there I was, paying overhead on the clinic, losing money hand over fist, deferring every dollar I made back into the practice, while still being on the hook for our Victory Hospital ownership payments.

It was the perfect storm for complete financial disaster. My relationship with the landlord only exacerbated these issues. About three years earlier, the physician owners of the medical office building, who I had a good relationship with and who recruited us to the building, sold the building to the Senior Housing Properties Trust (Nasdaq: SNH), a billion-dollar real estate investment trust (REIT) from Boston. Little did I know, I was signing a deal with "the devil." Like always, I had the contract reviewed by our corporate attorney, which turned out to be a mistake. I should have sent it to a real estate attorney instead, as there was terminology in the agreement that would bind me personally to the lease no matter what transpired in the business or my life.

At this point in time, we ended up hiring the consulting auditor full-time to help run the practice and to correct the mistakes that were being made. She agreed to accept the job as long as she was named the CEO, taking that title away from me. For good or for bad, I didn't mind giving it up at all because I had never been involved in the business side of the practice in the first place. I was busy focusing on my patients and their outcomes. Meanwhile, the office manager who had been with us for nearly ten years couldn't take the idea of the auditor taking over as the CEO, so she left.

Our new CEO, Linda, immediately began making decisions to recoup lost income and to ensure compliance and an organizational framework that would allow us to return to financial stability. She was operating autonomously, as LeAnn had stepped away from managing the finances and operations of the practice in 2014 so that we could prepare for the birth/adoption of our new baby, Ava.

Ever since LeAnn had our first child, Alexa, in 2002, and then our second, Caden, in 2005, she began to feel as if God had put it on her heart to have another child. But this time she wanted to *adopt* one. But since LeAnn was already thirty-seven, I suggested she have one more biological child. Then, I thought, if we still wanted another, we could adopt later. Thus, we had Colton in 2010, who was a tremendous blessing in our lives, as all children are. He is creative and entertaining, undeniably strong-willed but also softhearted. I wouldn't trade having him for anything.

But strangely, immediately after delivering Colton, LeAnn told me she *still* wanted to adopt. While still in the delivery suite she told me, "Let's adopt a little girl." We truly love children, so having a fourth child was appealing to me too. So, when Colton turned two years old, we signed up with an adoption agency, the Adoption Law Network, and created a profile, which included writing letters to potential biological mothers who were looking to give their babies up for adoption.

At the time, I was forty-two and LeAnn was a year younger. We waited, waited, and waited. After a year and a half, despite eight hundred views of our profile, not one biological mother selected us. Perplexed by this, I began to read letters written by those mothers, who almost universally sought out parents younger than thirty-five years old with *no* children of their own.

In their naivete and youth, to them, I guess we sounded too old and too preoccupied with our other three kids to be ideal adoptive parents. We were disheartened by this, to say the least. But I told LeAnn not to worry, "It'll happen in God's time." We certainly had enough to do in the meantime, with our busy lives balancing work with all aspects of taking care of our children, helping them with school, sports, and other activities.

But one day, our nanny, Ashley, found out that her twenty-year-old cousin was pregnant and was planning to abort the baby, as she had no way to support it. She soon asked her cousin to consider giving the baby up for adoption to us as an alternative. LeAnn had never lost her strong desire to adopt and had prayed about it often. She confided to me that she asked God to either take it off her heart to adopt if there was no baby for us or to find the perfect baby; this was only two weeks before finding out about Ashley's cousin's pregnancy. Needless to say, we were both ecstatic when she agreed to keep the baby and allow us to adopt.

About two months later, when we found out it was a girl, LeAnn allowed me to choose a name. I chose Ava (Latin for *life*), because her biological mother chose life and she was breathing new life into our family. We knew, of course, that there was a chance the biological mother could change her mind. But LeAnn and I felt that, even if she kept the baby, we will have saved the baby's life. If that was our only role, we were fine with it.

Six months later, we were in the delivery suite when our baby, Ava, was born. LeAnn cut the umbilical cord, which is something that never happens for the birth mother. Ava was perfect and chubby. Her biological mother stayed true to her commitment to us; she didn't back out.

To this day, Ava's positivity, crater-deep dimples, beautiful smile, and bubbly demeanor light up every room. She is the sweetest, most helpful little girl. She is like butterflies and rainbows and sugar wrapped up in a cute little package. She is a true gift from Heaven.

Back at the practice, with LeAnn gone and despite Linda's efforts, we continued to be late every month with the clinic bills, including our lease payments. In an attempt to decrease our overhead, Linda found two tenants to sublease the majority of the remaining space that was unoccupied due to the departure of all but three of our physicians.

Meanwhile, the Esaote MRI machine that we had purchased in 2013 had not turned out to be the moneymaker that we had hoped it would be. In fact, it was totally useless. Despite our due diligence, the MRI never functioned properly due to excessive interference in the building's electrical system. This meant that the unit could not be used during a normal workday because it would require us to turn off the air conditioning!

We weren't sure how that could've happened. Prior to purchasing the unit, we had consulted with the landlord's engineer and the physicist for the MRI company, who jointly determined where we should locate the unit to ensure that it functioned properly. In fact, we had already paid additional money to the architect to redesign the clinic space because the original location chosen, per the building engineer, would have resulted in too much interference. So much for his advice. The end result was that we had a non-functional machine.

Moreover, as if having the electrical issue wasn't bad enough, there were other obstacles too. Though we had been told that the model we purchased could accommodate all body types and all sections of the spine, that turned out to be untrue. So, patients who were larger than normal or who needed a scan of their thoracic spine (midback) were unable to be scanned at all.

In the end, we had purchased a $750,000 dust collector! After consulting with our attorney, our CEO, Linda, insisted that the company take the MRI back and requested a full refund, but they refused to do so. To mitigate our losses, we found an outside buyer for the unit, but the MRI company blocked that transaction too, stating that such a sale was a violation of a non-compete clause they had in that location.

Meanwhile, in an attempt to offload our overhead, our plan to sublease our additional clinic space to other physicians also turned out badly. For one year, these physicians in need of space were blocked by the landlord from subleasing, which was a clear violation of our lease agreement. We were told that the space would only be released *if* we became current on our payments. It was a catch-22. We couldn't *become* current without the additional financial support from those subtenants. Although we had only been two weeks late on average, that was not good enough for the intransigent landlord. As a solution, they negotiated a settlement with us in which we would pay them $100,000 up front to clear the lease from our primary space, which would then allow us to sublease the remainder. We borrowed this money from LeAnn's mother and got current on our payments on a Friday at the end of August 2015. The landlord waited until the following week when the new month started, and then maliciously claimed we were late again! I was infuriated by this tactic and felt entirely taken advantage of, as if I was being cheated or tricked.

So, even after confirming in writing that they would release the space, they now refused to do so after already taking our money. We consulted four different attorneys and each one of them recommended we vacate the building and litigate. I didn't feel good about that idea. I knew that getting into a legal battle with a massive REIT was going to be a losing and very expensive battle even if we were right, but I'm not a lawyer. Ultimately, after hearing the same legal advice again and again, I conceded, believing that it must've been the best course of action. So, much to my regret, we left the building for another location.

Next, because we had stopped paying for the defective MRI unit, the MRI company sued our clinic; then we countersued. A local radiologist offered to purchase the unit at *half* the value. I resented his capitalizing on my misfortune by giving us a low-ball offer, especially because I had been giving him a ton of business for years, sending him most of our MRI studies, but despite my loyalty to him, he clearly saw an opportunity to benefit financially. I later learned that the MRI company had negotiated these terms *with* him. On the one hand, the radiologist could acquire a cheap unit for himself while the MRI company could get themselves released from litigation. The offer only stood if we dropped our lawsuit against the MRI company.

I told my lawyer that I was not in favor of this arrangement, as again, it felt as if I was being both manipulated and cheated. I felt that we should litigate and that our case could easily be proven in court. My lawyer disagreed with me and even yelled at me to "stop trying to be a businessman and just practice medicine!" I almost fired him for his comments but didn't want to make a legal mistake. He told me that he knew what he was doing and I needed to listen.

Again, I conceded. His grand plan was to sue the MRI leasing company instead of the MRI manufacturer, pitting me against yet another billion-dollar company. This didn't make sense to me at all. But again, I'm not a lawyer.

Meanwhile, back at our medical office building, we heard from other co-tenants that SNH (the REIT/landlord) had reportedly been committing common area maintenance (CAM) fraud. We were told that overhead from buildings they owned in other cities, including Austin, was being dumped on our San Antonio location. I was told several of the tenants planned to leave and others decided not to renew their leases. It seems that we were surrounded by unscrupulous businesspeople and others who were making our work lives impossible.

In the summer of 2017, we discussed our leasing dilemma with yet another attorney who recommended suing the landlord for the violation of our lease terms and for fraud. Unfortunately, our lawyer was not as sharp as the attorney for the building landlord. So when he attempted to argue our point at a hearing, he got his butt handed to him.

After getting embarrassed at the hearing, our new attorney recommended that we file for bankruptcy. So here I was, facing two massive companies in litigation. What a mess! And who was going to fix it? If only I had consulted a real estate attorney to review and amend my leasing agreements for the MRI and the medical office building, I probably would have never been in this position. I won't make that mistake again.

Our CEO, Linda, admittedly had years of experience running offices and saving failing clinics and hospitals like ours, but it seemed as if even she was losing control of the situation and overwhelmed by it. Meanwhile, what did I know about solving these legal and business issues? My specialty was patient care. Frankly, even if I *had been* interested in the business side of medicine (which I was not), I would never have had time to manage the clinic without compromising what I did as a doctor.

Yet people always criticize doctors for not having any business acumen. What they don't understand is that physicians certainly have the intelligence, but just don't have the training, time, or skillset to do both well. You can either run the business well or practice medicine/surgery well. Something has to give.

After going through this experience, I think the most important thing to consider is the cost of your clinic space and the people who are hired to run it. First of all, keep your practice small. Hire great staff. It's better to have a small staff of great employees than a lot of bad employees. Often out of consideration of cost, administrators of practices pay lower salaries, but I believe it is much wiser to pay more and to have less staff who actually work hard. I also recommend contracts between physicians and their groups follow industry standards from the beginning. It is impossible to carry another physician's overhead. It's hard enough to cover your own. Everyone has to earn their keep.

Regarding lease terms, make sure you sign the shortest lease possible. Read the lease yourself, but also have a great real estate attorney review every detail of the contract and try to add an out in case you face financial difficulties or have a career-ending event. The landlord will expect you to pay the entire term of the lease, even if you vacate early. It's better to pursue legal action in the civil system than to allow the issue to go to bankruptcy court where a judge has full discretion to control your every asset. They're not all honest, and many are biased toward attorneys they've known for years. It's a bad position to get yourself into.

Chapter Thirteen

Et Tu

With litigation pending, the writing was certainly on the wall that we needed to extricate ourselves from the lease and move out of our office building ASAP. While searching for an alternate location to set up our clinic, I found a medical office space that was available and ready to be occupied. Upon further inquiry, the leasing agent asked me if I was part of the orthopaedic group that was leaving their current practice. I found the question strange, so I probed further.

It turns out that my colleagues and "close friends" at our current practice had been planning to abandon me and our practice (without notifying me) to set up a clinic of their own. I also found out they had also gone behind my back to ask for individual insurance credentialing through our credentialing coordinator in the clinic. Clearly, they were lining things up to be ready to practice independently. I didn't so much mind that they wanted to leave. It was the *way* they went about it, secretly planning, conspiring to take advantage until they were set up to walk away. I was hurt and furious.

What perturbed me the most about this discovery was that *they* were the primary reason I began to expand our clinic in the first place. In fact, my initial plan was to stay a solo practitioner. Eloy and I had committed to each other that we would never add any other providers to the clinic because very few people have the same perspective on patient care that we did, but I took a chance with these guys because two of them served in the military with me and one of them had become my very close friend from our first deployment to Iraq together. I struggled for years to help build their practices at my own expense, and now they were secretly leaving my practice without my knowledge.

I was furious, yes, but more than anything, I felt betrayed and used. On top of cashing out our kids' college savings plans, I had not taken a salary from the practice for two years. I had funneled every dollar of profit I made from the hospital (the one year we made a surplus) back into the practice to carry the overhead that, in part, was exorbitant because of *them*. For these guys to now stab me in the back after all I had done for them and their families was staggering.

The emotional cut was so deep that it's hard to describe. What made it particularly painful was the fact that each one of those guys considered themselves strong Christians. My closest friend of the three rationalized it by trying to say he told me. He never did.

What he did say is, "Maybe I should join another group to earn more money." It was a passing comment. It certainly wasn't, "I'm leaving without warning, and I'm taking the other guys with me."

He also tried to say that all of the marketing was focused on spine surgery, which was *very* far from the truth. In fact, our practice was primarily focused on orthopaedic surgery generally. Because I was so busy, I didn't need to market. When I spoke to LeAnn and Linda about this, both were incredulous and equally angry. Financially speaking, we were losing about $100,000 each month carrying the physicians in the practice. Yet we were willing to gut it out and continue to struggle alongside them until we were all in a better position financially. That's what friends do for each other, right?

Beyond my personal feelings, the main problem I had was that I was the only one responsible for the debt, as the sole owner of the practice. They had "no skin in the game" and clearly were not bothered at all by walking away, leaving me hold holding the proverbial bag.

A group decision was promptly made between me, Linda, and LeAnn. We would allow them to leave the practice, but on our terms—based on the contracts they signed. We set up a group meeting where I explained to them that I have found out their plan, and I was granting them their wish. Each of them had different contractual obligations to us and different minimum timelines to separate from the practice.

We held our end of the bargain and followed those minimum timelines stipulated in our contracts. They were very upset because it didn't give them the exact amount of time they needed to have all of their insurance contracts in place. They would later tell people in the community that they were kicked out in the middle of the night without warning.

The good news for me though was that I no longer had to carry their financial weight around my neck. I didn't have to feel guilty about separating them from the practice. Two out of three of them never exerted themselves enough to make a profit for the clinic, but I felt obligated to them as their friend to continue to help them build a practice and to make it successful. LeAnn and I decided the best route to take was to focus on what I did best and what we were most effective delivering, and that was taking care of spine patients. We knew how to run an efficient and effective spine practice and that we could count on my work ethic to make it successful.

Around the same time, in fall 2015, Victory Hospital filed for formal bankruptcy. Andrew and the owner of Victory Hospital, Bob Helms, had a falling out over unpaid bills and sued each other. Because Bob knew that I was the consultant for Andrew's implant company, when Victory filed for bankruptcy, he made me a third-party defendant, as if I had anything to do with their contractual agreements with each another. Bob was well aware that I was advising Andrew, but he also knew that I had no vote either in his hospital or in Andrew's companies. Luckily, I consulted with one of Andrew's attorneys, who brought the company agreements to the bankruptcy trustee to prove that I had no vote when it came to the implant pricing or any of the operations of Andrew's companies. He was also able to prove that Bob was well aware that I was consulting with the company as the CMO, as we had discussed it openly on previous text messages. I was immediately dismissed from the case.

Over the next two years, both LeAnn and I became increasingly skeptical of Andrew and his business practices. There was a buzz in the medical community that some doctors and administrators at Forest Park Hospital in Dallas were being investigated for alleged kickbacks. I knew that Andrew was affiliated with the hospital but had supposedly cut ties with them years earlier. I didn't think it was relevant until things started to change at TSM.

When Victory Hospital collapsed, multiple doctors stopped using the company's implants, leaving only a few surgeons still on board. whereas before there were up to fifty surgeons, or at least that's what Andrew said.

When it was obvious that Victory was failing, Andrew had refocused his attention on building his next venture, NextHealth—which, mentioned earlier, included a network of toxicology labs and compounding pharmacies. He had created this company with the other executives from TSM, *excluding* me.

Despite TSM's struggles (and NextHealth being in its infancy) I was hearing that Andrew was throwing lavish Christmas parties and giving elaborate gifts to the employees of NextHealth. He and Semyon were also jetting off on private planes to Puerto Rico to "expand NextHealth's businesses." (They both reportedly purchased grand homes there, complete with helipads.) Needless to say, the implant company began to tank.

With all that was happening in our medical businesses, LeAnn and I looked for opportunities to diversify *out* of medicine. For example, close friends of ours wanted to start an oil services company. The problem was that they didn't have the money to make it happen. We decided to invest a significant amount of money for the start-up costs and to become equal partners in their start-up.

Over time, the company unfortunately floundered as oil production in America was facing challenges from OPEC (Organization of the Petroleum Exporting Countries). The company *appeared* to be making slow and steady progress, but our financial troubles forced us to request our investment back so that we could use it to cover our debts and bills. We had used most of the money returned to us to do just that but still had about $200,000 left over. In the end, we learned it was best to "stay in your lane." It is best to do what you know best and have a natural gift for. We weren't familiar with the oil industry, so it was hard to contribute or to help the company grow; this distance from the industry ended up being to our detriment, and we were about to learn this lesson more than once.

In 2016, we met a guy named Prince Alex Tannous. We were told he was a prince from Dubai. LeAnn was introduced to Alex at the Horseshoe Bay Country Club by mutual friends who were credible businesspeople in San Antonio. One of them was an attorney we knew through mutual friends; the other was the son of the Jaffes, a well-known real estate development family.

When they first met, Alex shared with LeAnn that he owned a company in Dubai that manufactured and distributed juice drinks and other beverages. LeAnn eagerly called me over to meet him. We immediately started talking about a hobby that I had developed called the OsteoCorps. It was a STEM-based educational comic created to teach kids about their bodies, science, and the arts. I hoped to encourage kids to pursue careers in these subjects.

Toward that end, as I told the Prince, my OR team, and I would actually dress up as the superheroes and supervillains pictured in my comics and visit schools around the city to highlight how exciting learning could be. I had even envisioned one day having a healthy nutrition line for kids based on my educational characters.

In what seemed like fate, "Prince Alex" showed me press releases, Internet articles, and pictures of his drinks, including one that really intrigued me—a Superman energy drink. According to him, he had been given a licensing agreement for the beverage by Warner Brothers.

One day, he asked me why I had never developed my own products. My answer was that I didn't have the money to invest in it.

He then asked me what I would do if money were not an object. My response was that, of course, I would produce and distribute a line of my own. He said that he could definitely help me do it and offered to use his manufacturing plant to make this dream a reality. It wasn't long after that that he produced a partnership agreement, giving my company, OsteoCorps, a 49 percent share of our new business, while his company, Avaline, took 51 percent.

Admittedly, I was somewhat suspicious of this overly generous offer, but I soon let down my guard as Alex's connections to businesspeople that I knew seemed credible. Indeed, one of our local marketing friends vouched for the Prince, assuring us that he knew the Prince's relatives in Lebanon, that they were "an honest business family."

Of course, we still did our best to vet his company by querying other businesspeople we knew, together with international attorneys, while also doing our own Internet searches, but we could find nothing that gave us any reason to question his legitimacy. Plus, the sheer volume of information "the Prince" showed us seemed to establish his credibility.

Ultimately, the Prince convinced us to take a chance and invest $233,000 into making my dream a reality. It was a big gamble, as it was literally the only money we had in savings. (Our friend Rod Batson, invested $27,000 so that he could be a 10 percent owner of our share of the company.)

As the partnership evolved, I had my comic book artist from Brazil create mockups for our character-themed juices, drinks, and milk products. We even conceptualized a tea, water, and energy drink line. We also created brochures for our new company.

In the midst of all this planning, what ensued over the next months was a series of meetings, phone calls, and exchanges of emails with packing plants, juice box manufacturing companies, and suppliers of dairy and juice products. We also engaged in multiple meetings with marketers who worked directly with a large local grocery chain.

The Prince even brought samples of juices for me to taste. Since I had grown up overseas and could distinguish what fresh mango from Asia tasted like, it seemed authentic to me. I totally believed the Prince was the genuine article. It all seemed to add up.

You likely know where this story is going: In the end, no juices were ever manufactured or delivered. Every time we became suspicious, Prince Alex would copy me on phony communication memos with a marketing director or a manufacturing plant in America that sounded like he was actually going to make it happen.

Admittedly, there were some warning signs. The biggest red flag was that Alex kept asking for more money for marketing, money that we didn't have. What happened to the notion that "money was no object"? I guess an even bigger red flag was the fact that he called himself a prince in the first place. I feel so stupid for trusting him. Anyway, we eventually realized that it was all a farce—except to us, it wasn't funny. When we demanded the products, he acted like he was going to deliver them but he never did.

This scheme he had perpetrated on us was devastating, literally the final nail in our financial coffin. We considered going after the Prince legally, but since he was from Lebanon (not Dubai), there was no easy legal recourse for us. Also, we had so many other ongoing legal issues to deal with that we decided to let God handle the Prince in his own way and to move on! After all, he had already sent our money overseas and he apparently had no money of his own. This "Prince" was nothing but a Prince of Thieves.

When I look back at what happened, it seems absurd that we would have ever trusted him. However, as I said, the amount of documentation and detail that he produced would have convinced almost anyone.

Our efforts to diversify outside of medicine fell flat both times (with both the oil company and with the nutrition line) so we decided to thereafter stick with healthcare. As they say, stick with what you know. I'm not saying it's only possible to stick with one revenue stream. I just think it takes a lot of effort to diversify outside of one's field of expertise. I know of physicians who became so frustrated with medicine that they switched completely to business, to real estate development, or to a different industry altogether. I'm sure with the average intellect of a physician, those things are possible. However, as with all businesses, it's important to have a complete understanding of the industry before diving in. I think obtaining an MBA would be tremendously helpful for physicians, in general, especially those who wish to be more business-focused or to diversify outside of medicine.

Chapter Fourteen
As Sure as the Pope Is Catholic

In December 2016, the Texas medical community was shocked when the investigation of Forest Park Medical Center resulted in a notorious Department of Justice court case against a group of allegedly corrupt administrators, marketers, nurses, surgeons, and pain management doctors.

They were all indicted for a $200 million bribe and kickback scheme. The operation was designed "to induce doctors to steer lucrative patients—particularly those with high-reimbursing, out-of-network private insurance—to the hospital," according to the *Dallas Morning News* article that featured the story. Most of the kickbacks were disguised as consulting fees or "marketing money" doled as a percentage of surgeries each doctor referred to Forest Park. In the end, fourteen defendants were convicted, sentenced to a combined more than seventy-four years in federal prison, and ordered to pay a total of $82.9 million in restitution.

Not surprisingly, Andrew was one of the defendants!

As I eventually learned, prior to partnering with Victory Hospital, Andrew and Semyon had worked with Forest Park, recruiting doctors and marketing services for the hospital, "scheming behind the scenes" just as described in the court case.

Andrew had tried to get me to go to Forest Park a decade earlier, but I had declined and was unaware of what was happening there. In any case, at the time the news of the indictments broke, Andrew initially blew it all off, saying it was all "nonsense" and that there was nothing for him to worry about. In fact, Andrew and Semyon, his business partner in every business and the Russian guy I met at Craighead's party years earlier, seemed unfazed by the indictments; although I don't know how it's possible not to worry about something like that.

Then, out of the blue, Andrew sent his executives to San Antonio to tell me that his implant company, TSM, was being closed. It seemed suspiciously abrupt to me. Why in the world would Andrew close a company that was still profitable? Everything he did happened so quickly, I just knew that something was awry. He also immediately fired the entire team of sales reps in San Antonio. Unfortunately, I had encouraged them all to take the job with Andrew, so I felt quite guilty as they now had no way to provide for their families.

At this point, with all of Andrew's erratic and destructive actions, I became suspicious that he had been doing something illegal in one of his businesses, which could also impact me and LeAnn. When I reached out to Andrew to ask him about why he closed the company, he stonewalled and wouldn't tell me anything. I then called a knowledgeable individual and asked him what he thought about Andrew's action to close the implant company. I specifically asked if he thought Andrew was moving money from TSM to make it look like it wasn't very profitable.

"F—, yeah, as sure as the Pope is Catholic!" he responded in a flash. So, just as LeAnn and I suspected, he agreed it was likely that Andrew was secretly moving money to his new company, NextHealth, to pad his pockets. LeAnn asked if he thought we should sue for the money Andrew owed us, and he answered we definitely should do so. He recommended we seek the help of a friend of his who was a great litigator and an honest guy, someone who would empathize with our plight.

Our association with Andrew had obviously been a total mistake. We had devoted so much time and effort building the implant company, TSM, with the hope that it would one day offer state-of-the-art products that would lead to a profit. I had put an incredible amount of effort into developing that line: as CMO, I helped find the products and identify manufacturers, recruit doctors, and advise on product efficacy, while also assembling reps and distributors.

While I did all this, working as hard as I did, Andrew dangled the promise that TSM might eventually get a buyout from a bigger company that would lead to stratospheric profits, a "liquidity event" that would solve all our financial problems. Clearly this was merely a ploy to fool us into helping him grow the company. Indeed, he dangled the carrot continually, telling us that a buyout was imminent. It would be, in his words, our retirement plan.

So, in 2016, while everything else was failing, with our medical practice struggling and our office space downsizing, we still held on to the hope that TSM would help carry us financially until Andrew pulled the carpet from under us. That dream was now dead.

At this point, with Victory Hospital bankrupt and TSM closed, we were totally disgusted with Andrew and his highly publicized indictment. Clearly, we had been fooled into trusting someone who had betrayed our trust and broken multiple laws.

We weren't going to give up on our investment in TSM, not without a fight. To dig into what was really going on, our attorney, Lenny Vitullo, requested financial records from TSM, as we had not seen any statements for a year. This period of time coincided with the upswing in Andrew's NextHealth Laboratories. We suspected that money was being moved from TSM to NextHealth—a money-siphoning scheme to keep the implant company less profitable, while hoarding all of the profit in NextHealth so the executives and the owners could reap the financial rewards by minimizing their overhead.

Later, when NextHealth was indicted, we heard from a previous employee that its executives would hire prostitutes and fly them on their plane all over the country, giving lavish parties—all at the expense of the companies Andrew owned. It *was* the healthcare version of *The Wolf of Wall Street*!

Our lawyer recommended that we mediate with Andrew and Semyon in order come to a settlement for the money that was owed to us, as LeAnn's family trust had invested in TSM. When the money was siphoned off, it essentially stole profits that were owed back to the trust of what was estimated to be millions of dollars.

Andrew and Semyon scheduled the meditation in Dallas, but once we got there after a four-hour drive, Andrew and Semyon walked out on the meeting, completely disinterested in negotiating at all. I'm sure they found it amusing that they had wasted our time traveling to Dallas only to walk out on us. Before they left, they had refused to acknowledge that they had moved money and even suggested that we had something to do with the failure of the implant company. Clearly, despite my being the CMO of TSM, neither LeAnn nor I had any vote in the company, nor any management input whatsoever. Andrew knew this and so did his attorneys.

In January 2017, in order to save the practice, LeAnn, who was busy taking care of our new baby, Ava, was forced to return to the office so she could properly handle all the business dealings and our legal issues too.

Our CEO, Linda, clearly needed help and direction. LeAnn's management would allow me to redirect my energies to the actual practice of medicine, focusing solely on patient care. However, because, as the CEO, Linda had made all the business decisions for our practice between 2013 and 2017, she was now entirely entangled in the legal conflict with SNH, being deposed and attacked by the opposing attorneys.

With lawyers gunning for her, she panicked and broke under the pressure. It was just too much for her to handle. So, in the interests of her mental and physical health, she left amicably for a less stressful life in January 2017, just as the legal battle between my clinic, OSI, and SNH and Key Finance was warming up. I understood her decision. I would have left, too, if I wasn't the one who had assumed all the risk for everyone else's decisions as the owner of the practice.

Around the same time, UnitedHealthcare filed a suit against Andrew's company, NextHealth, accusing the Dallas-based laboratory network of a $150 million scheme involving kickbacks to physicians and other providers for overpriced and unnecessary drug and genetic tests. *Oh my!* Another lawsuit against Andrew. We had apparently been working with a total crook.

UnitedHealthcare even alleged that sales consultants from Andrew's company offered fifty-dollar gift cards to people who provided urine samples in a Whataburger bathroom as part of the "wellness study." Multiple toxicology labs around the country were sued by the major insurance carriers for alleged "fraudulent billing" and, because the number of dollars involved was so high, the federal government became involved. The legal heat was turning up for Andrew and Semyon in every way possible.

This new lawsuit between UnitedHealthcare and NextHealth unfolded while Andrew and Semyon were still under federal indictment for their involvement in the Forest Park Hospital scandal. Once that happened, it created more urgency on Andrew's and Semyon's parts to settle the lawsuit between us. They realized that our allegation that they siphoned money out of TSM created bad optics for them. As if they needed any more bad publicity. UnitedHealthcare also went after multiple doctors who had invested in the NextHealth labs legally, threatening to kick them out of network (and actually doing it to some) despite it being illegal to remove doctors from an insurance network for referring outside of the network. Doctors just typically give into this despotism by doing nothing. I don't know of any doctor who has the financial means to fight a giant like UnitedHealthcare or any other big insurance carrier.

So, in April 2017, TSM reached out to us to settle the case. We were finally able to obtain financials that proved that they had, in fact, siphoned millions of dollars away from the implant company to the laboratory company to maximize their profitability while leaving us out. We came to a monetary settlement of a little more than $1.5 million. Although the details of the settlement were confidential, it became public record in legal proceedings that followed later when the judge ordered the information be disclosed.

At the time, our attorney, as good as he was, made what turned out to be a significant miscalculation in his petition to the court: he wrote the papers as if I were *personally* suing Andrew and his partners at TSM. He explained that he felt it would add more impact if the case ever went to trial to have an individual name versus a business name as the plaintiff. We don't understand legal semantics, but as things turned out, this technicality created an opportunity for misinterpretation later. The plaintiffs should have been LeAnn's family trust, not me! I was merely a trustee and had no personal rights to any of the settlement. So, the money went back to pay off the trust's debts, including its investment in Victory Hospital. The Victory debt repayment would still take another three years to pay off. This small detail in the petition wording would come back to haunt us later.

In July 2018, as reported by the *Dallas Morning News*, Andrew and Semyon were then arrested for smuggling medical marijuana from California to Texas. The feds seized their shipment and immediately charged them with drug trafficking, adding to their incredible record of misdeeds and illegalities. There they were, facing federal healthcare kickback charges and a $150 million fraud lawsuit. Yet they apparently couldn't stop themselves and were in even deeper trouble now.

Their flippant attitude about the Forest Park indictment changed dramatically, because the feds now had them on two cases, one more extreme than the other. They were going down for sure now.

They knew it and, knowing Andrew, he was going to craft an evil scheme to get out of it.

As he had proven, he was brilliantly devious and crafty. And I'm sure he used all the skill he had to figure out how to get back at us for suing him and anyone else he could throw under the bus in order to lessen his sentence. I was an attractive target as one of the busiest spine surgeons in Texas. Andrew knew it would be a huge feather in someone's hat to indict a busy spine surgeon like me. The truth was not going to matter. Just getting out of trouble, by any means necessary, was the name of the game.

Around June 2017, with the TSM lawsuit settled, LeAnn was back to the drawing board, trying to figure out how to save our sinking ship and help us get out of debt. Without the legal differences yet settled between our medical office building landlord (SNH) and our MRI leasing company (Key Finance), we moved out of that complex into a much smaller, more affordable office building.

LeAnn met with our attorney, Peter Stanton, to strategize next steps to fight the two pending lawsuits. As I explained earlier, Stanton had been intimidated by his defeat at the initial hearing with SNH and had already conceded the battle. So, he had LeAnn meet with another lawyer in his practice, Ron Johnson, who was a bankruptcy specialist.

Ron explained to me and LeAnn that SNH was a multibillion-dollar company out for blood. They were seeking a payout from us of $3 million for "violating" our lease (i.e., vacating the premises without paying out on the full six years remaining on the lease). SNH's lead attorney, Joe Davis, supposedly made the comment to Peter that they were going to make us "bleed money."

But we still felt like we had a case against them for the violation of their sublease agreement with us and for the CAM fraud we believed they were committing. One of my main issues was the personal guarantees I had signed when SNH bought the medical office building. I was not made aware by any of my attorneys that I should have signed the lease agreements, and every contract for that matter, with my name *followed* by my company title.

    This is because personal guarantees bind you personally, even if you are signing for an LLC. These personal guarantees can be a financial disaster for an unsuspecting physician. This commonly happens in real estate leases and in physician-owned hospital deals. Many of those deals are merely a real estate scam where the general partners (not the physicians) flip the land and building to a REIT upon completing construction for an immediate financial gain, while putting the doctors on the operations side of the ownership, obligating them to operating costs, and long-term leases under a personal guarantee. Many medical office building leases and business investments require the physician to sign a personal guarantee, hooking the physician personally into the debt even if the business goes belly up. The businesspeople file bankruptcy and walk away. Meanwhile, the doctor is on the hook until the loan is paid off, even when the facility is closed or defunct. We paid a giant monthly note on Victory Hospital for five years *after* it was closed! Always try to avoid that issue by signing your named followed by your title (as the CEO, president, CMO, etc.) in the company you are investing through. In general, a physician should never sign a contract without their lawyer reviewing it and without their company title following his/her signature, or they will be personally liable.

    In the midst of this conflict with our clinic landlord, we also had to figure out how to resolve the MRI situation. Six months prior, our specialist primary clinic attorney had a motion for summary judgment hearing with a local judge against Key Finance, a leasing company for the MRI Company. In the court, by his own admission, our clinic attorney spent fifteen minutes explaining our position, while the opposing attorney for the MRI leasing company spent *an hour and a half* presenting her argument. He felt that was all the time necessary to get his point across.

However, the judge decided in Key's favor, tapping us with a $400,000 judgment, the entire amount of the lease, including interest that would have accrued if we had paid it off over the term of the lease. As you can imagine, I was furious about this turn of events. Our attorney had been a great attorney for us, but earlier he yelled at me for disagreeing about the lawsuit against the leasing company in the first place. As I had assumed and the judge decreed, it made no sense to sue the leasing company when the people who were responsible for the malfunctioning MRI was the *manufacturing* company that was let off the hook.

Oddly enough, for a period of eight months after Key Finance won the motion for summary judgment, we didn't hear back from them about collecting the judgment or structuring a payment plan. Our attorney called several times, but their counsel never responded. We suspected that they were waiting to see what was going to happen with the SNH lawsuit.

Finally, around August of 2017, we heard back from the Key Finance attorney. Together, we set up a plan for LeAnn to begin payments on the ruling, which required us to pay back approximately $400,000. Simultaneously, we continued negotiations with SNH.

How were we going to float all this overhead? LeAnn's initial impulse was to sell her family's lake house (an investment property purchased by her family trust). By doing this, she could use the proceeds to pay off SNH and relieve pressure on the Key Finance tab, but the problem was that we could not control when a home buyer would come along. Also, our clinic attorney, Mark Weitz, wisely reminded us not to use the trust assets to pay off a personal debt.

Overall, despite the weight of the large payment installments to Key Finance, LeAnn worked that debt into her budget with terms that we thought we could afford. But our solvency depended upon our landlord, SNH, accepting a reasonable settlement. As we found out, SNH was not willing to budge and continued to threaten us with their absurd demand of $3 million.

After making several payments to Key Finance, LeAnn realized, in consultation with Peter and Ron, that there was no hope for getting a reasonable settlement with SNH. They were just too "bloodthirsty." So, Ron strongly recommended that we file and declare bankruptcy in order to create a fresh start.

Never in my wildest dreams had I imagined that I would be in this position. At this point, I had been practicing as a physician for twenty years; and I had demonstrated an exemplary record of financial and surgical success. Indeed, our practice had been booming from 2005 when it opened to 2013. And yet, here we were with a practice that was imploding.

With no other option, I reluctantly filed the papers for bankruptcy in January 2018. And as always, while all the legal maneuverings were happening in the background, I let LeAnn handle the business and legal issues while I just kept my head down and focused on taking care of my patients.

With the loss of the big office, our legal issues, and the bills that ensued, LeAnn's family trust—BHT (which her parents established in 2009 for LeAnn and our kids)—became our flotation fund, keeping our practice afloat. Fortunately, LeAnn had managed her trust as an investment vehicle and had done very well with it, while all *my* investments had failed because the practice and hospital overhead were so high.

This operational burden for most physicians is sinking their spirits and their practices. As I said earlier, the insurance companies dictate our fees (i.e., reimbursements that are hardly enough to cover costs to practice). This is why doctors are leaving medicine, talking their children out of the profession, retiring early, and generally disenchanted with the practice of medicine.

In 2021, the physician burnout rate was reported to be 42 percent based on a report by Medscape in their survey of over 12,000 physicians in more than twenty-nine specialties. Female physicians report a 51 percent burnout rate, even higher than their male counterparts. Although the COVID-19 pandemic added to their stresses, 79 percent of those physicians reported their burnout began before the pandemic. The top reasons for their burnout include too many bureaucratic tasks, too many hours at work, lack of respect, and insufficient compensation.

Surprisingly, those physicians who work in a healthcare organization report the highest level of burnout. This proves that corporations' dictating physician responsibilities and work environment do a poorer job than when physicians are at the helm. Yet, doctors are joining these organizations because they simply can't afford to practice on their own. Reimbursements have declined so dramatically that they see it as the only way to continue practicing medicine.

This is a sad reality for the most educated people in the country, whose lives are devoted to improving and saving the lives of others. In the same survey, increased financial compensation to avoid financial stress was listed as the number one solution to reduce burnout. And, even more concerning, was the finding that 89 percent of physicians surveyed reported being depressed. This disturbing trend is not going to improve unless we fix the issues stealing the joy and life from physicians.

Clearly, LeAnn's skilled attempt to resurrect my practice was a losing battle. She explained, "Look, I need to create a new practice, one that I control financially. For the past three years, other people have been making bad decisions, which have put us into massive debt. I'm not going to assume that debt. Those weren't my decisions. I'm not going to put my family trust at risk like that, but I'll start a new practice and come back into the office to run it."

LeAnn decided to develop a practice focused solely on spine surgery. We named it SASpine—Surgical Associates in Spine. (Conveniently, for the previous fifteen years, our office URL was SASpine.com, which allowed for continuity.) LeAnn and the new practice administrator, Liz Knight, who had expertise in revenue cycle management, built the administrative side of the practice from the ground up. LeAnn purchased an entirely new electronic medical records system, billing software, and a practice management system. She, with Liz, also established new contracts with the insurance companies, created a new business with its own tax ID number, and even revamped the phone system. Additionally, she purchased some of the equipment and furnishings from the previous practice based upon an appraisal to determine fair market value.

Meanwhile, going from a staff of 105 down to twenty-five, we brought into the new streamlined practice just our primary pain management doctors, our neurologist, our physical therapist, plus a few new mid-level providers.

Everything in the office had to be done by the book. No mistakes were made (or so we thought), and so began a new chapter of our lives, one in which our new medical practice grew...but our legal entanglements only worsened.

Chapter Fifteen

In God We "Trust"

In September 2018, we realized that our initial team of attorneys (Stanton and Johnson) for the bankruptcy and litigation against SNH and Key needed reinforcements. The situation was getting too complex, and there was no case law precedent for it.

Mark, our trusted clinic attorney, did one great thing for us: he referred LeAnn to one of the best bankruptcy attorneys in the country, Eric Taube, who was based out of Austin. When she asked Ron Johnson about Eric, he concurred that, even though he would probably lose a client, that "Eric Taube is the *best* bankruptcy attorney in the country." LeAnn knew she had to retain him. He is a Vanderbilt grad with a booming voice, imposing demeanor, and confidence that is unmistakable.

When LeAnn approached him about weighing in on the case, he almost turned it down. He is typically strapped with huge high-dollar corporate cases that pay more and are more worth his while. But after reviewing our lawsuits he decided to help—as God would have it. One thing was clear from the beginning for Eric, and that was that we should *never* have filed for bankruptcy. He explained to me and LeAnn that bankruptcy gives the judge sole authority over your fate. He felt with LeAnn handling all the financial issues through her family trust (although she wasn't obligated to since they weren't trust debts) that it would have been better to battle it out with SNH and Key in the civil court system and to keep covering the costs of the practice as she was doing. Unfortunately, it was too late, and we were in a bind that he had to unravel, unpackage, and get us out of.

Indeed, in a series of strategic maneuvers, the attorneys for Key Finance, SNH, and even the bankruptcy trustee (the attorney appointed by the court to ensure the creditors are paid accordingly) teamed up against us, shooting every missile at us possible.

At the beginning of the bankruptcy in the fall of 2018, the attorney assigned by the court to be the trustee hired two lawyers to be part of his team. What surprised me was that the trustee was not an unbiased liaison of the court—this attorney was assigned to collect money, wherever possible, for the creditors.

The trustee assigned in our case, his team, and the attorneys representing the landlord SNH and Key Finance teamed up with one another to go after me, LeAnn, and her family trust. In their pursuit of money, they were alleging all types of nefarious acts that never occurred.

One of the trustee's attorneys was a sniveling, high-water-pants-wearing weasel of a lawyer who decided he would go after LeAnn by suing her personally and even her family trust. He had the nickname "Curly" because he looked and acted like one of the Three Stooges (although he looked more like Larry than Curly).

Curly was missing one key point: The bankruptcy had nothing to do with LeAnn's family trust or with her personally. She wasn't the one who filed for bankruptcy. They had no right to go after her or her family trust, but they wanted to fill their greedy clients' paws with money, even if they weren't entitled to it. They may have been funny looking, but this wasn't funny at all.

We had the constitutional right to file for bankruptcy, but our adversaries assumed it was not possible that I was *legitimately* filing. They were convinced that I had hidden resources (i.e., that I had moved money around to avoid paying my debts and had even manipulated LeAnn's family trust to hide money). In short, they set out to prove we were committing fraud, alleging that I was the "mastermind" behind the trust and just "pretending" to be financially overwhelmed.

They subpoenaed *everything*—my phone(s), our computers, our emails, and all of our company records, but because they were only able to request up to five years of records, the end result left them with only a partial picture of our businesses, the trust, and our financial history. In an effort to undermine our credibility and demonstrate the extravagance of our lifestyle, they obtained a video that was produced by a friend of ours, which pictured our two homes (including the homestead I bought while active duty and another that LeAnn's family trust purchased).

Of course, they conveniently neglected to point out to the judge that these two homes were owned by two different entities (i.e., that I only owned *one* of them, while LeAnn's *family trust* owned the other). And I was the one being implicated. It didn't matter that I bought that home after saving every penny I earned by working more than one hundred hours per week. I had obtained an interest-only loan for the property and had put almost every dollar I ever made into that home as a real estate investment for my family's future.

In any case, the opposing attorneys led the judge to believe that I owned both homes and that I was craftily manipulating the bankruptcy law. *As if!* In short, they used every bit of propaganda they could to paint me as a devious fraudster who was shirking his financial responsibilities. Moreover, they implied that I was using my wife as a scapegoat for my own supposed misdeeds. And the bankruptcy judge, Judge Craig A. Gargotta, bought their depiction of me hook, line, and sinker. It was clear that he was biased in each hearing (and there were many). I must say that things were looking bad for us because our attorneys, Ron and Peter, had a hard time isolating each allegation and systematically disproving them. Between my practice and LeAnn's family trust, there were multiple entities that confused the opposing counsel. They assumed that I owned everything and was hiding my assets in LeAnn's family trust. Everyone refused to believe the trust generated its own wealth, because they were not privy to documentation going back to the creation of the trust and the companies it invested in more than five years earlier.

We knew we would eventually win because the truth was on our side, but the road to getting there would be long, emotionally arduous, and costly.

In the fall of 2018, soon after hiring the hotshot bankruptcy attorney Eric Taube, LeAnn received a frightening email from Richard Roper. He was the attorney who had cleared me from any wrongdoing during the investigation into Allure four years earlier. Roper followed his call with an email that shocked us all: "Steve is being targeted for federal indictment and I cannot represent him!"

As you read in Chapter One, my world came to a screeching halt. For starters, at the time LeAnn got this message, she was driving in the car with our oldest daughter, Alexa (who was then sixteen years old). LeAnn immediately called up Richard and asked what this ominous message was all about. He didn't have all the details yet but it had something to do with my old arrangement with Julia Eller, dating back to the indictment of Rooney and Allure in 2014. It had been four years since then and nine years since I worked on implant designs for Allure in 2009. Roper later explained he was conflicted it was because he had represented Andrew in the past.

While thinking about what to do, LeAnn, who had a lot of friends who were attorneys, thought to herself, *I have to call Mike McCrum*, a well-respected criminal defense attorney with whom we had mutual friends. Instantly Alexa exclaimed, "Mike McCrum! I *love* Mike McCrum!"

Amused, LeAnn thought it was impossible that Alexa would know who he was. But Alexa insisted she did know Mr. McCrum and that he was "awesome!" Alexa, who is an aspiring attorney, explained that while interning over the summer in the district attorney's office, she sat in on a murder trial. McCrum was giving closing arguments in the case. Prior to McCrum's closing argument, Alexa was convinced the defendant was guilty. But after McCrum was finished with his argument to the jury, my daughter was convinced his client was innocent.

In short, McCrum had made a huge impression and his name stuck in her memory. Never did she imagine that McCrum would become a household name at our dinner table months later and ultimately a guardian angel to her parents.

McCrum was not only famous for his talent as an attorney but also highly respected because of his integrity. He was a former police officer, federal prosecutor, and strong Christian. He had a track record of success in criminal defense that was uncommon, even when facing large corporate entities like BP Oil.

After a grueling day in the operating room, I opened my email to read Roper's message with the news of my pending "indictment." My heart dropped. That night, I sat in my bedroom feeling helpless. I thought that I had already been exonerated from any wrongdoing four years earlier. Why in the world was it coming back to haunt me yet again? Honestly, at this point, there were so many people attacking me simultaneously that I really had nowhere else to turn to *but* God.

All my life I have tried to meet God's expectations of me while also being immensely strengthened by my faith, but it seemed all my accomplishments came with extreme hardship and a heavy emotional toll. Nothing came easily, and it felt as if LeAnn and I were sinking into quicksand, dragged down by all these unfair legal maneuverings. In addition to prayers, we absolutely needed the best legal help possible.

Although McCrum was in high demand, we had a mutual friend who called him on our behalf. McCrum immediately called LeAnn and agreed to accept our request to represent me. The first thing Mike did was call Roper, who disclosed the nature of the accusation to McCrum. Apparently, Andrew was behind the resurrection of this old investigation.

As it turned out, Andrew needed to curry favor with the feds by cooking up several schemes to try to implicate us. Each was well laid out and sprinkled with just enough truth to make it sound credible, though it was all really a pack of lies. As LeAnn would often say, "It takes a lot to get into the criminal mind of Andrew Hillman." Indeed, Andrew had a way of making everything he did seem honest and ethical. We never knew the extent of his treachery until I filed for the bankruptcy in 2018. It was the perfect opening for Andrew to attack. With the bankruptcy, we believe Andrew decided he could make even more accusations that tied us to bankruptcy fraud as well. The settlement money he was forced to pay LeAnn's trust could easily be misrepresented as payments that I was hiding from the bankruptcy trustee. Only, it wasn't my money. It merely added yet another accusation to try to pin on us. The crazy thing is, the federal investigators seemed to believe what he was saying, and—according to witnesses they interviewed—the feds had named Andrew as the source of their suspicions.

The first attempt to frame us, as part of an attempted plea bargain, was to allege that I received kickbacks from Julia at Allure. It had been nine years since the last time I consulted with Allure, and we had *already* provided documentation that proved otherwise many years prior. I thought that this issue had been laid to rest, but because Andrew was familiar with the details, here was this old information against us. I guess the statute of limitations was irrelevant to the investigators. LeAnn had collected all the files from that time period after they were sent back by Roper, but it had been so long that she couldn't remember where they were in the move from San Antonio to Houston.

When McCrum explained the accusation to us, we were less than shocked that Andrew could be going down this road. He would do anything to hurt us in order to minimize his own jail time. Of course, he knew full well the allegation of kickbacks with Allure wasn't true. One thing I learned about this absurd process is that proven criminals can get a plea bargain if they turn on others they are legitimately connected to. They can even get away with lying; they can claim an illegal act happened with someone to prove this purported affiliate's guilt if the investigators/agents listening to this story are susceptible to these lies. The liars are already in trouble and apparently won't face any further penalties for stories they make up, as long as the agents can't prove they are lying. I'm told that their penalties will only become less harsh if their accusations against another result in a conviction. So, crooks know to say whatever they can to lessen their sentence. The agents then take what they hear and start investigating, bringing people like me under a cloud of suspicion even if initiated by lies. Although our attorneys told us that fabrications could result in heavier penalties for people who lie to the investigators, as long as the agents can prove they were being lied to, that clearly wasn't likely to be the case with Andrew.

After all, in the beginning, every business arrangement we had with Andrew was completely legally vetted by our attorney. Additionally, Andrew supposedly consulted multiple attorneys, and he was always very careful not to trip over Stark or Anti-Kickback laws or commercial bribery laws. In fact, he talked nonstop about "compliance."

So, on the surface, he seemed just as concerned as we were about following the rules. It's what caused us to drop our guard and to trust him in the first place. He was a really great con man: he treated you like his best friend, showered you with compliments, and seemed to be as devoted a father and husband as I was. Luckily, because we were always committed to following the rules (especially coming out of the military), we always double-checked everything we did—not only with his in-house counsel, but, more importantly, with our *own* independent healthcare attorney as well.

To sum it up, there were no illegal arrangements between us and Andrew, or any other business for that matter, including Allure and Victory Hospital. The problem was *he* was a crook and a liar. His arrangements with us were legal, but they were one-sided. He made sure he was the one in the driver's seat and profited immensely from every deal at everyone else's expense. He moved money from company to company, playing a shell game, so his investors made little profit and he rode the companies to the bank.

As I think about it now, I think Andrew is some kind of sociopath and narcissist—a lethal combination. He didn't care who he stepped on as he climbed to the top. So everyone's back was a stepping-stone to financial success for him, but of course, the reason he was about to be shipped off to jail for sixty months was because he got greedy and eventually very sloppy.

Looking back, I always wondered why Andrew hired a CEO for all his companies instead of assuming that role himself. I figured it was because he needed someone to delegate responsibility to since he was so busy running his "sixty-plus" businesses.

In truth, he needed a fall guy, someone who would take the risk at the helm, unwittingly being backstabbed by the owner himself. A red light should have gone off when I saw that every move he made in company operations seemed convoluted and unnecessarily complex.

The reason he operated this way became quite apparent when he began trying to get a plea bargain for his crimes. What better person to implicate than the person he just had to settle a lawsuit with for stealing money—yours truly!

As stated earlier, Andrew was now being investigated for multiple federal offenses. The most egregious offense was conspiring to juggle the proceeds of various healthcare entities, including his pharmacies, resulting in $150 million in fraudulent billings to government and private insurance programs. Among other alleged fraudulent activities, the pharmacies were accused of paying illegal kickbacks to doctors and others to generate prescriptions, self-funded patient copays to dupe auditors, and misbranded drugs.

Though Andrew was perilously threatened by federal charges, he apparently still had time to let his vendetta against me fester. He obviously resented us for being forced to settle that lawsuit for $1.5 million.

With Andrew on the defensive and under considerable risk of doing jail time for at least one of his federal indictments, he had the incentive to methodically manipulate our past business dealings in an effort to implicate us and to lessen his sentence. Andrew would be planning a strategic game of chess, attempting to be several moves ahead of us for months. He was going to try his best to drag us down with him.

At this point, between our bankruptcy proceedings and now a federal investigation, we had a total of four lawyers handling our legal battles, including McCrum and Taube. Meanwhile, our adversaries were armed with a total of at least six lawyers. This included two attorneys on the bankruptcy front, two representing the MRI company, and two advocating for the medical office building.

Together, they were aggressive and doing everything they could to create a narrative that wasn't true. Although we had total confidence in our new and improved legal team, we were fighting battles on multiple fronts, and the pressure was crushing us, especially LeAnn, who was saddled with handling all the legal details. She stayed up late at night and spent most days poring through her computer, printing documents, going through emails, and reproducing the events of the past ten years in writing to show the truth. She had a filing system that served her well.

LeAnn and I were fully prepared to prove our innocence in

the bankruptcy case, but the opposing counsel was now alleging that we committed bankruptcy fraud, which turned a civil issue into a federal one. To top it off, we were now in the midst of a federal investigation in which allegation after allegation was being hurled against me, all thanks to Andrew. I hadn't done any of the things alleged, *not one*. I felt like Joseph in the Bible, falsely accused and facing persecution for crimes I didn't commit. I tried to keep reminding myself of Isaiah 54:17: "No weapon fashioned against you shall succeed, and you shall confute every tongue that rises against you in judgment. This is the heritage of the servants of the Lord and their vindication from me, declares the Lord."

Although I referred frequently to the Bible for inspiration and peace, I still lost many nights of sleep with all this happening. The problem was, with patients to take care of daily, and a wife and kids to provide for, I didn't have the luxury of wallowing in misery, or giving up, or even spending much time figuring out how to defend myself.

As I said, this left the burden of most of the legal meetings and collection of records to LeAnn and our attorneys, with me weighing in on the rare occasion when I was free. My problem was, I had little to do with any business arrangements, financial matters, or company decisions. LeAnn and our previous CEO had handled it all. In the beginning, our attorneys kept referring to *me* for information in the bankruptcy mess; and I kept referring them back to LeAnn. Yet nobody believed that LeAnn was really in control of all our finances and operations of the practice, not even our own attorneys, in the beginning.

I didn't even know what our assets *were*. I know that sounds ridiculous, but I didn't have time for that. I was working twelve- to sixteen-hour days. LeAnn handled all our business affairs and was truly the real brains behind the operation. (I was just the brain performing the operations.)

It took a while, but eventually our attorneys came to the realization that it was LeAnn whom they needed to work with when it came to clarifying every and anything legal. It was much harder to convince the opposing counsel of this fact. Even the lead attorney for Key (who was a woman) refused to acknowledge LeAnn was anything more than a doctor's pretty wife. It was demeaning and chauvinistic, much less from another woman, but they continued to assume and even say that *I* was the one who set everything up and was using my wife as a diversion to that fact. It couldn't be further from the truth.

In our dealings with Andrew over the years, there were many occasions in which he told us he purged his records frequently. He recommended we do the same. We did not agree with him. In fact, we felt that keeping all emails, files, texts, and records was the best way to prove compliance; and we were right. It turned out that every email ever sent, every text, every file, contract, agreement, everything, was still in our computers and on our phones dating back to 2005.

When our computer and phones were ultimately subpoenaed by the opposing bankruptcy trio (the bankruptcy trustee and his attorneys and the Key and the SNH attorneys), it actually proved we were, indeed, telling the truth. LeAnn loves the story that our bankruptcy attorney, Ron, tells about his wife reviewing every single one of my phone records, texts, search history, and pictures. Mind you, I had more than 20,000 pictures and 20,000 emails and texts to review, so it was a lengthy process.

As Ron tells it, in his thirty years as an attorney, he had seen multiple clients' emails and phone records and never in his career had he seen so little incriminating evidence; there wasn't even a mistake on my tax returns.

Indeed, after reviewing the totality of my messages and emails, Ron told LeAnn that his wife really came to love and respect me because my messages were always positive, including frequent Bible verses I sent my kids and wife to uplift their days; there was no profanity, and no nude pictures, nor inappropriate messages anywhere to be found. He said she thought I was "the next closest thing to Jesus," clearly partly in jest, but it was nice to know my lawyer knew my heart as a faithful husband and father, a loving son and brother, and a dedicated surgeon.

Needless to say, I was happy Ron knew I wasn't whom I was being painted out to be. I just had to prove that to Judge Gargotta. But from my observation in the courtroom, it seemed as if the opposing counsel had totally won over Gargotta, who seemed to believe everything being dished up by the opposing counsel.

The only negative thing they could come up with was a video of our home in San Antonio, as if that had anything to do with our need to declare bankruptcy. Yes, I had a big house because I worked hard and saved every penny for the down payment and my monthly mortgage payments. There was no crime in having a big house! As Ron often said, "So what?" But as we learned, the opposing counsel did everything possible to impugn anything they could about me to influence the court in a negative direction. Since they couldn't attack my character, they were now going after the house, my only asset!

During one of the days in court, they were alleging that the move to Houston resulted in the abandonment of our homestead in San Antonio. This wasn't true, because at the time of the filing we still lived in San Antonio, making it our homestead. A homestead is protected by very strict laws, making it almost impossible to take away your primary home, even in bankruptcy.

    LeAnn and I were called to defend this homestead to prove we hadn't abandoned it. During a break in the hearing, I just happened to go to the restroom at the same time as the attorney representing SNH (the landlord). I was so annoyed by their gross distortions that I told the lawyer, "I'm so glad I don't have your job. I would feel horrible about myself if I had to lie every day just to make money, even stooping so low in an attempt to steal someone's home from them." He stared at me without a word, as if he knew I was right. I wonder how these people can feel good about their jobs, but they were ruthless and inhumane, doing anything they could to win.

Chapter Sixteen

Out of the Frying Pan, into the Oven

Getting back to the allegation of kickbacks, I'm sure Andrew was banking on the idea that so much time had passed, we had not kept our files and the proof of the diligent work I completed with Allure. But as I've said, LeAnn had kept every previous form of communication. Who keeps emails and phone messages that far back? We did, though we almost lost some key materials. At one point, when we were moving, LeAnn had instructed one of our movers to "get rid of everything left in the garage." She believed there was nothing of importance left over.

Serendipitously, our friend Jordan, who was clearing out the garage, had the intuition to verify if the box was actually trash. When he saw a random cardboard box in the garage, he thought it looked important. So instead of tossing it, he brought it to LeAnn in Houston. Thank God!

When LeAnn got the box and looked inside it, it was a gold

mine. It contained all the files and documentation related to my consulting agreement with Allure: old drawings I made of spinal implants, time sheets, invoices, emails, and corporate documents dating back to 2008.

Thereafter, LeAnn stuck it in her office closet and thought nothing of it. Fast forwarding to her first conversation with McCrum, she recalled having the box and pulled it from the closet, explaining, "I actually have all the documentation right here." She promptly sent the entire file to McCrum.

As the federal investigation instigated by Andrew proceeded, one person after the next began contacting me, informing me that they were approached by two investigators, one from the Department of Labor and the other from the FBI. They had gone around San Antonio asking questions about me, my family, and my practice.

They went to my sister-in-law's practice (she's a dentist) and passed out their cards explaining they were conducting an investigation, within earshot of her staff and patients. They went to my elderly widowed mother's house, asking questions about me and my business.

The investigators questioned my older brother, colleagues, and anyone they could, including my equipment reps in the operating room, looking for any information on me that was incriminating. They repeated Andrew's lies as if they were true, alleging that I had received kickbacks, to see if people would say negative things about me. Most everyone had nothing to say because there was nothing negative to say. A lot of people were too intimidated to speak openly about how they felt about Andrew. Yet, the investigators were still unconvinced of my innocence.

But because we were able to provide McCrum with all evidence needed in order to dismiss the allegation related to Allure, he provided it to the assistant U.S. attorney and the investigators. We thought we were in the clear, but Andrew wasn't finished yet.

When the initial Allure allegation failed, Andrew came up with a new one: he alleged that I had accepted kickbacks for Department of Labor (DOL) patients while working at Innova. I heard this lie was corroborated by the chiropractor whose business I declined, the one who referred to surgeons as "cutters." In my entire career as a spine surgeon, I had only performed surgery on a grand total of six DOL patients! Four of those came from the clinics owned by Dr. Craighead, the zany chiropractor I discussed previously. I never got paid a dime for two of the four surgeries I performed—let alone did I receive a kickback of any kind. They actually owe me money.

As I stated earlier, I never even used Allure implants on those patients. I just consulted to improve and create new designs and had the documentation to prove it. In any case, once we showed our documentation of the paltry number of DOL surgeries I performed (along with the minimal revenue earned), the federal investigators realized there was nothing to pursue.

Once again, the records that we kept delivered me from another false allegation.

LeAnn was more determined than ever to beat Andrew at his elaborate game of deception. It was, in her mind, like a game of chess, and we needed to anticipate and block his next move. We got to the point where LeAnn would produce the documentation proving an arrangement was legal even before the next allegation surfaced.

As we soon discovered, the third allegation from Andrew was that I had an illegal marketing arrangement with Victory Hospital. That was the type of allegation that ultimately led to the indictments and convictions of the Forest Park doctors. However, as I mentioned previously, we were at no risk of violating those laws because we made sure our healthcare attorney either crafted every arrangement we had or, at a minimum, signed off on them. Marketing was a big one. There are very specific rules that have to be followed.

Firstly, in order to have a legal joint marketing agreement between a doctor/clinic and a hospital, each entity must split the cost of marketing fifty-fifty. For example, if marketing costs $50,000, the clinic has to cover $25,000 and the remaining $25,000 comes from the hospital. Also, that $25,000 from the business entity/hospital cannot go to the doctor or to his clinic. It must go directly to the vendors.

Additionally, we hired a third-party marketing company, which handled all the marketing arrangements for us. The final requirement to make joint marketing legal is that all advertising must represent the logo for both entities. We met all of those criteria, so that allegation fell flat as well.

As always, LeAnn had kept meticulous spreadsheets of what she paid versus what the hospitals paid, in addition to photo renderings of the actual billboards purchased showing both companies represented. Undeterred, Andrew kept creating new scenarios, and the investigators kept indulging his fabrications. It was as if they wanted him to be right. At this point, the investigators had spent so much in government resources on us, I guess they felt they had to find *something*.

The fourth allegation that one of the federal agents repeated, further impugning us in the community, was that money was traced from various accounts into Andrew's account and then funneled into ours. The amounts were between $100,000 and $200,000. But what happened in reality was that we asked the parent company, TSM, for a loan to pay taxes for the shifty accounting they were performing, which led us to being taxed significantly more than expected.

LeAnn obtained a promissory note from our healthcare attorney accounting for the money borrowed from our partners, worth $750,000, with terms including interest that we would be committing to. But Andrew seemed overly relaxed about the repayment, which was atypical for him. To be sure everything was above board, LeAnn was very aggressive about repaying the money in a timely manner. She dealt directly with the CFO to ensure it happened correctly. We discovered later, Andrew's laissez-faire attitude was likely a set up. It seems he was planning to use the loan as a kickback allegation if anything went awry for him and he needed something on us that he could bargain with.

Ultimately, he could act as if the loan wasn't a legitimate loan at all; it was a kickback and this information could potentially be given to the feds for leniency. When the agents alleged they traced money from one account to the next, we uncovered his scheme. It finally made sense to LeAnn why he paid out the loan in small chunks versus the $750,000 in full. According to one of the people the federal agents interviewed, the agent alleged payments we received were a veiled kickback. Andrew had created an indistinct money trail, as most criminals do. Andrew was such a crook that he set everything up in a way that could be proven legitimate or he could twist some details and use it to point the finger at others, if he was ever busted for breaking the law. He failed again as LeAnn was able to prove up the loan agreement and payback amounts. She even had wire confirmation of the smaller amounts that totaled up the $750,000 to true up the loan amount and correlated it with the promissory note.

When the federal agents saw this very clear money trail from Andrew to us was in fact legitimate, and not what Andrew had told them, they moved on to the next allegation he drummed up. For whatever reason, they kept chasing his allegations as if they were hoping one of these far-fetched lies was true. They seemed intent to continue digging until something turned up.

The next (and most absurd) lie Andrew concocted was that LeAnn and I headed a crime family, which included my widowed seventy-five-year-old mother and two brothers. (I should note that my older brother never worked with me at all!) Years prior, my mother and younger brother purchased a brace company, but it went bust due to poor reimbursements and limited business. What's worse is that Andrew obtained $25,000 worth of braces from them and never even paid them for the inventory. Now he was sending the feds after them. This guy was willing to stoop to the lowest levels, even resorting to attacking my elderly mother living on social security.

The ridiculous allegation was that a former lieutenant colonel in the Air Force had turned into a crime boss! This was hilarious. Such a baseless assertion died soon after we showed emails dating back to 2008, in which I advised everyone at the clinic against ordering medical devices for government patients from my mother's or brother's companies.

When Andrew's previous allegations failed, he decided to attack his own marketing arrangement he had established with LeAnn to build his company, Health Crave. He claimed that the payments he made to LeAnn were illegitimate and that she didn't perform any marketing function. This was patently ludicrous. Countless observers in San Antonio would have remembered the numerous billboards, commercials, and radio ads LeAnn had placed to market the company, and she could prove it with comprehensive records showing the hours billed, the marketing efforts made, and the receipts for everything from business cards and website costs, to paid invoices for events produced and marketing employees hired. She also had emails dating back to 2011, proving that she had told Andrew that she couldn't possibly build *his* company's brand for free. Andrew agreed in writing that he would pay her for her services. (And by the way, LeAnn wound up spending far more on marketing than she was paid, thinking it would be beneficial in the end, which it was not!) All this was more than enough evidence to prove, once again, that Andrew was a total liar.

One of Andrew's most desperate attempts to implicate us was when he convinced the bankruptcy attorneys that the money we won in the settlement against him/TSM was being hidden from the bankruptcy court. In other words, he claimed that settlement money (40 percent of which went to the attorney) was being hidden. Thus, we were committing bankruptcy fraud. (By the way, Andrew didn't even pay the remaining installments of the money owed to us.) He even alleged that my brother was hiding the money *for* me.

Financial records subpoenaed from us and my brother disproved this farce. Yet as you can see, Andrew kept sending the investigators down new rabbit holes, and they kept looking. Andrew even tried to accuse one of my best friends, Rod Batson, of hiding money for us by saying that we had Rod buy our cars in his name! When he was questioned by the investigators, Rod asked, "If my cars really belonged to the Cyrs, then what cars do my wife and I own? And why are they in my garage?" Then Andrew's lawyers tried another tactic, asking how much we paid our nannies. Why? Because Rod's nanny and our nanny were sisters. So, the insinuation was that we were over-paying the nannies to hide money. All this was laughable. The whole investigation into our finances had truly gone from the ridiculous to the stupid. Remember, these expensive investigations are funded by taxpayers' money. It is a total waste of our government's resources that spanned years. Talk about fraud, waste, and abuse.

As I look back on it now, I think Rod's candid testimony convinced them that there was no aspect of our finances that weren't on the up and up. Ultimately the investigation into our business dealings was dropped and no charges were ever filed against me, but a lot of damage was done in the process. Believe it or not, I am grateful they listened to Rod. I do think they were really trying to get to the bottom of the truth.

Unfortunately, when federal investigators realize there is no case against you, they seem to disappear without considering what harm their investigation may have caused to your reputation. They do not go back to clear the name they spent months tarnishing with innuendo and leading questions. The more than three hundred people they interviewed never got a follow-up message confirming my innocence.

In fact, shortly after Rod's meeting with them, the lead investigator told Rod that she had concluded that "Dr. Cyr was a noble guy," and that my biggest problem was going to be the lingering bankruptcy case that was still pending. I'm glad she came to that conclusion, but I sure wish she would have told that to the people she questioned throughout this investigation.

She did explain, however, that the attorney for Key, Leslie Luttrell, had it out for us and was doing everything she could to win her lawsuit against us. Indeed, Luttrell would continue to lead the charge of continued false claims against us and attempt to smear our name, locally and nationally.

In fact, one day I received a call from a pain management doctor whom I referred patients to in Houston. He called to ask about family trusts. He told me that he had read an article about me and my family that alleged we had a self-settled family trust. I was shocked by this revelation and asked him to send me a copy of the article, published in *Forbes* on April 15, 2019, outlining the bankruptcy case we were going through. It was titled "Third-Party-Created Trust May Be a Self-Settled Trust and Included in Bankruptcy Estate in Cyr Case." The careless bankruptcy attorney who authored the article, Jay Adkisson, enumerated every allegation as if they were truths, not claims. What he didn't know or acknowledge was that each allegation *was* slowly being disproven in court.

Yet he claimed that LeAnn's family trust was self-settled. That meant that it was funded by her and therefore illegitimate, which meant that the assets were fair game to the opposing bankruptcy trio. In our view, Adkisson had no basis for the comments other than false allegations and certainly didn't understand the details of the case, which was still ongoing. Though the financial odds were stacked against us, LeAnn and I were confident that the truth would be revealed, as long as she could afford our legal defense.

The writer drew the conclusion that our "goose was cooked," because all of the allegations had to be true. His presumption was, of course, entirely incorrect and not based on fact, but it didn't stop him from writing this absurd article that circulated nationwide. I strongly suspect the Key attorney had something to do with passing the case to him as one of her serial attempts to bash us publicly and to create bias against us in the court.

I must say that the rumors circulating around the investigation and the *Forbes* article did a lot of damage. It was impossible to keep our bankruptcy a secret, as all the misinformation spread rapidly throughout San Antonio, which is really a small town, despite it being the seventh-largest city in the United States. Friends from all over called to ask if we were okay. It was terribly embarrassing. Our clinic volume dropped 30 percent. A lot of people thought I had been run out of the city and was a crook or a fraudster. It was a very demoralizing time.

We came from humble beginnings and had spent years trying to give back to the city, spreading blessings by funding multiple charities, sponsoring children for camps, visiting schools to teach kids about STEM, chairing fund-raising galas, you name it. Through it all, we strived to be positive role models in the city we called home.

But now all that had been tarnished by a couple of money-hungry, self-serving attorneys and further boosted by erroneous reporting in a national publication. After our request for a retraction from *Forbes* fell on deaf ears, LeAnn struck back at the attorney for his inaccurate article, filing five grievances against him in every state he was licensed. News of our grievances were picked up by multiple news sources via press reports nationwide, leaving the writer with his own public relations issue to deal with.

Chapter Seventeen

Vindication

As our bankruptcy case lingered on, LeAnn was spending money hand-over-fist for our defense. Our attorney Taube was brilliant... but expensive. And the stress of it was taking its toll on LeAnn. She couldn't sleep. She was visibly distressed daily. She was losing her hair due to the stress she was under. In short, she was miserable. I felt so bad for her.

But she is a tough woman. And it was inspiring to see her pull it all together when the kids were home. After all, she had to be a mom, and we did not want our personal struggles to negatively affect our children. Our kids had just made a huge transition, and each of them was being affected differently by the move to Houston.

Our eldest, Alexa, was a star pupil and still competing in pageants. Her final pageant—the Miss Texas Teen USA competition—took place in the heat of the turmoil during her junior year in high school. Moreover, she was busy preparing applications for top-tier colleges and studying ferociously for the SAT. LeAnn has a special expertise in career counseling from her early career and used that knowledge to help Alexa prepare her applications.

Every day, LeAnn would shake off the anguish of dealing with the lawsuits, subpoenas, and allegations and switch into mom mode to help the kids handle their personal issues. But it was extremely distracting and emotionally draining for her.

With Alexa, it was college applications and traveling to universities all around the country. Caden, on the other hand, really struggled with the move to Houston. He was going into his freshman year and left behind very close friends in San Antonio. He was not happy about the move and needed extra love and support during the transition.

Colton had his own struggles. He was diagnosed with a vestibular disorder that affected his coordination and vision, making it difficult to focus in school. Fortunately, that little guy is resilient. He began physical, occupational, and eye therapy at the age of four and continued that rigorous schedule in Houston as well. LeAnn worked tirelessly to support his therapy while trying to get the teachers and administrators at his new school to understand and accommodate his educational needs. They didn't seem to get it, adding further to our frustration.

While LeAnn was handling complex legal matters, she would frequently get calls from the principal that Colton was sent to her for misbehaving. It turns out that he did not understand the instructions or couldn't see the board. When he asked for clarification, the teachers were reluctant to give it. He would roll his eyes and get sent promptly to the principal for "blatant disrespect." They cared more about his eye-rolling than the bullies who were constantly picking on the new little kid with glasses. That was frustrating. At least Ava was so young that she required almost no additional academic or emotional support. She did need mommy time though.

But there LeAnn was, saving our family from lawsuits and federal investigations—all while trying to rebuild our businesses and constantly switch into loving, devoted mom mode at the drop of a hat. She had to, as she describes, shape-shift constantly between businesswoman and concerned mother. She is a remarkable woman.

She balanced her responsibilities masterfully, but the stress made her defensive, suspicious, and angry. What did fall to the wayside was LeAnn's social life and our joint charitable efforts. LeAnn had always had a strong core of close friends who she saw frequently. Also, we had been both actively involved in charities and the social scene in San Antonio. But at this point in our lives, there was no time left for relaxation or for anything social. Our sole focus had to be on our children and our legal battles.

I handle stress by staying busy at work then turning it off when I get home. LeAnn handled it by switching into problem-solver mode. It's a good thing that LeAnn is strong, because that amount of stress and pressure would have broken almost anyone. Fortunately for us, she's a fighter, *and* the truth was on our side. We believe God is too; and He had protected us on so many occasions before. I referred nightly to Psalms in the Bible. It gave me peace to read about David's unwavering faith amid his struggles. I read consistently to reinforce my faith and was reassured by several passages. Some of the many verses that gave me peace were as follows:

Psalm 27:1–3—"The LORD is my light and my salvation; whom shall I fear? The LORD is the stronghold of my life—of whom shall I be afraid? When the wicked advance against me to devour me, it is my enemies and my foes who will stumble and fall. Though an army besiege me, my heart will not fear; though war break out against me, even then I will be confident."

Psalm 91:1–16—"Whoever dwells in the shelter of the Most High will rest in the shadow of the Almighty. I will say of the Lord, 'He is my refuge and my fortress, my God, in whom I trust.' Surely he will save you from the fowler's snare and from the deadly pestilence. He will cover you with his feathers, and under his wings you will find refuge; his faithfulness will be your shield and rampart. You will not fear the terror of night, nor the arrow that flies by day, nor the pestilence that stalks in the darkness, nor the plague that destroys at midday. A thousand may fall at your side, ten thousand at your right hand, but it will not come near you. You will only observe with your eyes and see the punishment of the wicked. If you say, 'The Lord is my refuge,' and you make the Most High your dwelling, no harm will overtake you, no disaster will come near your tent. For he will command his angels concerning you to guard you in all your ways; they will lift you up in their hands, so that you will not strike your foot against a stone. You will tread on the lion and the cobra; you will trample the great lion and the serpent. 'Because he loves me,' says the Lord, 'I will rescue him; I will protect him, for he acknowledges my name. He will call on me, and I will answer him; I will be with him in trouble, I will deliver him and honor him. With long life I will satisfy him and show him my salvation.'"

Psalm 109:2–5—"For people who are wicked and deceitful have opened their mouths against me; they have spoken against me with lying tongues. With words of hatred they surround me; they attack me without cause. In return for my friendship they accuse me but I am a man of prayer. They repay me evil for good, and hatred for my friendship."

Isaiah 41:10—"So do not fear, for I am with you; do not be dismayed, for I am your God. I will strengthen you and help you; I will uphold you with my righteous right hand."

One of the main accusations that the *Forbes* article harped on was the issue of our homestead (primary home), a 7,000-square-foot house that was my pride and joy, because I saved every penny for the down payment while I was active duty. It is a beautiful home with a castle-like facade that encircles a pool in a center courtyard with a waterfall into the pool. It had even won the People's Choice Award in a Parade of Homes the year it was built in 2007.

No doubt, the creditors wanted to take this home and sell it off as an asset; and they used every angle they could to get the court to turn it over to them. They even claimed that we abandoned our homestead when LeAnn and the kids moved to Houston—long after we filed.

But according to the bankruptcy "snapshot rule," homestead is determined at the time of filing (i.e., where you are living at the time the paperwork is submitted). Moreover, even after LeAnn moved to Houston with the kids, to get away from it all, I never left the home. Since my primary clinic was in San Antonio, I was still staying there three to four days per week, so I couldn't leave if I had wanted to.

Because our daughter was Miss Houston Teen the previous year (while a San Antonio resident), they also tried to use her Houston title as proof that we lived in Houston (though we didn't). Toward this end, the Key attorney, Luttrell, was even willing to damage our children's futures by sending subpoenas to both pageant systems Alexa competed in (USA and America), even though LeAnn offered to send them whatever records they needed to avoid that. The repercussions of these legal ploys were that pageant leadership became aware of our bankruptcy and the accusations of fraud, dashing my daughter's hopes of ever being crowned in those systems going forward.

Luttrell's despicable tactics pushed LeAnn to her limit. She was absolutely livid that Lutrell would have the audacity to involve our children in this mess. We were both amazed she would stoop to those depths. She had really gone too far, and the judge was enabling her to do it by not putting a stop to her antics. This brought the fierce mama bear in LeAnn to the surface, as she expressed a new level of anger that I had never previously seen.

At this point, she went after Leslie Luttrell, the Key attorney, filing grievances against her with the State Bar of Texas. The situation was clearly escalating, and everyone involved knew it. At one point, Judge Gargotta strangely ruled that the homestead was no longer protected. It was a landmark gaffe and error on his part. I think he just wanted to throw the opposing counsel, who he was obviously fond of, a bone if possible, no matter how absurd.

Prior to that, Eric Taube had done a masterful job at each hearing, forcing the judge to rule on the law without opinion or bias, so that he ruled in our favor on every issue. Our attorneys were therefore shocked at his decision, as was most of the legal community. The aftermath of this ruling created a mass panic in the estate planning community, as everyone was equally shocked with the unusual ruling on the bankruptcy judge's part. In fact, according to our estate planning attorney, it spurred a Texas bill to make sure the property code and the tax codes had the same wording to avoid another bad judgment in the future (the technicality he used to justify his decision).

We appealed the decision, the result being that the appeals courts quickly overturned the bankruptcy judge's flawed ruling, stating the judge had focused on "style over substance" and that his ruling was in error. In short, our homestead exemption was returned to us, keeping it as a protected asset from the bankruptcy proceedings.

Although we had jumped through this legal hurdle, LeAnn had a bad premonition that more obstacles were soon to follow. In fact, as she warned Eric and Mike, she was relatively confident that Andrew and the conniving counsel would join forces to defeat us. And she was right.

As LeAnn suspected, they next alleged bankruptcy fraud! Though such an offense couldn't be further from the truth, it made no difference to our ruthless adversaries, who had an agenda to win by any means necessary.

You may recall earlier that I referenced the lawsuit against Andrew and his partners in which our attorney styled the (lawsuit) petition using my individual name as the plaintiff, instead of LeAnn's family trust. The problem with using my name was that any settlement money naturally had to go back to the trust, since the ownership was purchased *by* the trust, not me. Lenny explained that he styled it the way he did to appeal to a jury if the case were to go to trial—they would have more sympathy for an individual than for an entity.

Due to this technicality, the creditors and their attorneys claimed that the money actually belonged to me and it was an attempt to "hide" the money to avoid paying personal debts, but I was not legally entitled to the settlement proceeds, as it wasn't my investment. (In fact, the company agreement between the trust and Andrew's company had been drafted by Andrew's attorney,

Nick Oberheiden, who knew very well that the investments were owned by the trust.)

But the creditors and their attorneys—jumping on the nuances in the petition—alleged foul play. Of course, we weren't attorneys. We just provided information to our lawyers who we trusted to make the call on those types of issues.

Everyone involved knew that the investments belonged to the trust and that the respective money stolen was trust money. So upon settlement, the money must be returned to the investing entity, which was the trust. In retrospect, the petition should have had both names on it—so that Lenny had the individual effect needed for a jury and the correct entity could be paid without scrutiny. But—at the time—we had no idea that we would end up in bankruptcy court one day and this would become a point of contention.

At this point, Eric filed a compelling motion for summary judgment proving the funds belonged to the trust, not to me. Our opponents could manipulate the truth, but the facts were clear. There was no fraud. Only the trust was entitled to the settlement and the settlement proceeds went directly to the trust creditors. That was the nail that sealed the coffin on all the allegations against us. The attorney for Key Finance, Luttrell, had pulled out all the stops. On the heels of the closing of the investigation with the Department of Labor, it seemed as if she was waiting to see if there was any merit to these new allegations. Bankruptcy fraud is a federal offense and would fall under the bankruptcy judge's jurisdiction if it were true. Fortunately, with the motion for summary judgment showing there was no fraud, the creditors and their attorney finally gave in and agreed to settle the case.

In March of 2021, after three years of legal battles, with the opposing counsel finally on the ropes, LeAnn decided to agree to a reasonable settlement. She had endured the attempt to penetrate her family trust, the *Forbes* article, and all the mental anguish that went along with it, not to mention our legal fees, which were astronomical. In the end, we had won each battle, but at a significant emotional and financial cost.

As she reflected on it, LeAnn felt that the opposing attorneys' ferocity went way beyond the proper limits of zealous advocacy. Maybe they believed what they were alleging, but they sure didn't seem interested in the facts.

We heard later that the primary antagonist in our bankruptcy battle, Luttrell, had been up for consideration for a position as a federal judge but was passed over, in part, perhaps, as a result of LeAnn's grievances filed against her. Although we don't wish for negative things to befall others, I can't help but to feel a slight sense of vindication that she wasn't rewarded for her mercenary approach and dirty tactics with a lofty position that would put others under her sole control and discretion as a judge. What a scary thought!

We believed in our heart of hearts that had we continued to fight, we would have prevailed on the few issues that were still pending, but at an exorbitant cost. Our attorney, Eric, was definitely the hero in this situation. He had wisely recommended settlement so we could move forward with our lives. Looking back, I can see that he literally saved us from the bankruptcy vultures and greedy businesspeople. His talent in bankruptcy law is unparalleled.

Mike McCrum provided our documents to the federal investigators and quelled any further investigation into our business dealings. A true blessing to us, he never charged us more than our initial engagement fee. In his defense of our case, his integrity and compassion were evident all along the way.

To us, his Christian faith was evident in the way he practiced law. To thank him, we gave him a sculpture of Saint Michael defeating Satan with his favorite verse inscribed on a plaque: Isaiah 56:1—"Maintain justice and do what is right, for my salvation is close at hand and my righteousness will soon be revealed."

In addition, Rod Batson, my longtime friend and one of the equipment vendors, had come to our defense in a way that only a true friend could. He truly knew us and our business dealings and impactfully cleared our names so the investigators could see the truth. Without his coming to our defense, we may have had many more issues to deal with. Thankfully, the investigators finally saw the truth.

Others also defended our name and deserve credit for being honest instead of just assuming our guilt because allegations were raining down upon us. As we had discovered, few people stand beside you when that happens. I am grateful to those who stood for me and the truth.

One of them was our healthcare attorney, who has been a true lifesaver from the time we first met him in 2008. His faithful guidance and attention to all compliance reviews and proper contracts have kept us safe. We are eternally grateful for him.

In addition, our CPA, Norbert Gonzalez, has done a masterful job ensuring our finances and taxes are properly handled ever since we started our practice in 2005.

As for Andrew's fate: As a co-owner of Hospital Business Concepts, Andrew would ultimately plead guilty in October 2018 to conspiracy to pay and receive healthcare bribes, and he was sentenced in December 2019 to sixty months. But because he was sentenced to prison with COVID-19 in full bloom, I hear that he was slated to spend most of his sentence at home under house arrest. We were recently told, however, that he never returned to prison and was working as a paralegal (go figure) and selling COVID-19 tests. I guess you can't keep a good man down.

We have since moved on in every sense of the word. Traumatic as it was to be falsely accused by a pathological liar like Andrew and his cronies, we had to draw a line in the sand and say *enough!*

I left this entire legal nightmare beyond frustrated with the snakes in government-and-insurance-managed medicine. Through it all, I learned some very difficult lessons, and I have benefited from mistakes I hope to never repeat and that other doctors can avoid.

Throughout my life, I've seen institutional corruption and the corrosive nature of jealousy and greed. I've weathered reversals of fortune, bad business decisions, and the threat of unscrupulous people who attempted to destroy us. Indeed, I wasn't aware that I was partnering with criminals and liars! I also never expected people that I trusted, including fellow physicians, to betray me, but they did.

Sure, I have a responsibility for the decisions I made, driven by my desire to focus on what was best for my patients. Maybe I should have been more involved in the business side of the practice. But honestly, I couldn't have done that administrative work and still maintained the quality of care.

If I were to do it all over again, I would still never compromise my patients to be more involved and successful financially as a businessman. The fact is, we as physicians are vulnerable prey to the system. The only way to protect yourself is to be armed with a clear understanding of the Stark and Anti-Kickback laws and Racketeer Influenced and Corrupt Organizations (RICO) laws, and to seek certified healthcare, real estate, and corporate attorneys for advice at the appropriate times. More importantly, follow their advice and read every contract. Medicine is not what it used to be. We have far more to worry about than malpractice lawsuits. Have a contract for everything—including between you and your physician partners—that protects you from the potential collapse of a practice.

Try to avoid bankruptcy at all costs. It puts all the power into the hands of a bankruptcy trustee who will side with creditors and, even worse, a judge who may also be biased against you in favor of creditors. Bankruptcy fraud is a federal offense, and greedy creditors will do anything they can to get their money, including lie to get their way. Don't sign any contracts you haven't thoroughly read and reviewed with an attorney who is a specialist in that field.

But through all the challenges and stressors over a quarter century, God has guided and protected both me and LeAnn, strengthening us. My wife's attention to detail protected me, but our faith carried us both through very trying times.

Disgusted as I have been with insurance-driven medicine, I decided to forge ahead into a new specialty as a back-up to an insurance-based practice. So, in 2019, I began a two-year cosmetic surgery fellowship with the president of the American Board of Cosmetic Surgery, which I hope will also pave the way for an extended medical career. It certainly wasn't easy to relegate myself to the position of a student/fellow after more than twenty years in practice. But, I'm willing to do whatever it takes to provide for my family. I love spine surgery, but there are a couple of issues with it long term. I fear reimbursements will continue to decline and regulations and costs will continue to increase. Moreover, I don't know how long I can practice like this: long days that run into late nights.

Why do I say this? Because my primary career as a spinal surgeon with a focus on complex surgery requires arduous fourteen- to sixteen-hour days in surgery—a regimen that I may not be able to maintain for another fifteen to twenty years. Whereas cosmetic procedures, though requiring significant skill, are not so physically demanding; many of the surgeries last for a shorter period of time. Because these procedures are not insurance-funded, I don't have to deal with those insurance companies anymore! I refuse to be painted in a corner. My family's livelihood is at stake, and I don't trust the system or the direction medicine is headed. I love spine surgery and will continue to do it, as long as it makes sense. With cosmetic surgery, I can have the best of both worlds.

With my energies directed toward this transition, I completed my fellowship in February 2021 as the *world's first* orthopaedic spine surgeon and fellowship-trained cosmetic surgeon.

I should say that my passion for cosmetic surgery is definitely driven by my lifelong interest in aesthetics, fitness, nutrition, and health. Over the years, patient after patient asked me to consider taking a little bit off "here and there" or doing a "simultaneous tummy tuck" during my anterior approaches through the stomach to the spine. I've always loved cosmetic surgery as a discipline and its ability to both transform a person's appearance *and* their feelings about themselves.

During this period, armed with formal training in liposculpture and cosmetic surgery, I pioneered a new surgical technique called OrthoSculpt, a procedure in which fat is preferentially removed from the body to highlight a person's natural musculature and shape deep to the fat. This procedure, which requires an understanding of the muscle and bony anatomy of the extremities and torso, tapped into my extensive training as an orthopaedic surgeon.

I have thus been able to increase the anatomic accuracy and precision of current techniques, going beyond them to promise better (and safer) cosmetic results for my patients.

With a new dimension to my career, and our legal problems resolved, life has returned to normal, and I feel a sense of renewed energy and optimism. My cosmetic practice is blossoming, my spine surgical practice is booming, and our clinic is right-sized and run efficiently by LeAnn and her team.

Most important, LeAnn is happy and relatively stress-free while our kids are healthy and excelling in school. In short, all is well in the world. And I have a back-up plan for surgery that can carry me into my seventies, should I desire to keep doing surgery. But life is full of ups and downs. One of my realizations in life is that contentment is more important than happiness because it can be constant whereas happiness is temporary.

Chapter Eighteen
Beauty from Ashes

Isaiah 61:3—"...to bestow on them a crown of beauty instead of ashes, the oil of joy instead of mourning, and a garment of praise instead of a spirit of despair."

By spring of 2021, with our legal battles all behind us, all seemed to be going so *well*. But then on the evening of May 18th, there was an enormous thunderstorm in Houston with a tornado watch alert. I was scheduled to have left earlier that evening for San Antonio, as I had surgery there the next morning, but—because of the storm—LeAnn recommended I wait until the morning to leave.

That night, because of the tornado warning, I took the two little kids, Ava, six, and Colton, ten, into our bedroom, which is located on the ground floor. Meanwhile, I told Caden that he should go downstairs as well and sleep in Alexa's room since she was away at college. Caden didn't listen to me and slept upstairs instead.

At midnight, LeAnn woke me up because our home alarm went off. When I got up and turned off the alarm on the panel, I noticed the garage was signaling an error. On the way to the garage, I noticed that our central vacuum cleaners were running. I unplugged them because I couldn't figure out how to otherwise turn them off.

As I continued toward the garage, I heard Colton and Caden screaming in the front of the house. I opened the gate to see what was going on and Caden was yelling, "Our house is on fire!"

Apparently, during the electrical storm, lightning struck the house and it was now in flames. The impact of the thunder had set off the alarm, though I didn't connect the two facts at the time. I quickly ran back inside the house and grabbed our fire extinguisher. I ran upstairs toward the smoke but only made it to the third step before I was overcome by toxic fumes. It had only been about five minutes, but I couldn't see and I couldn't breathe. Even though I had been accustomed to wartime chaos, I had never experienced such immediate disorientation; the smoke was overpowering and caustic. Everyone was standing in the foyer trying to figure out what to save and what to do. The house was a lost cause. Realizing how dire the situation was, we all left the house immediately.

We called 911, and more than twenty firefighters showed up, their combined total taken from three fire departments in neighboring cities. As the team rushed into our home, we all watched in a state of shock.

As the fire grew larger and larger, with flames leaping from the roof and extending down into the heart of our home, I kept asking myself, *What's taking them so long to extinguish it?* It seemed like nothing was happening, despite their efforts.

On the outside of the house, the fire chief had a single fire hose directed toward the top of the house toward the flames. The tiles were flying off, left and right. Eventually, after four hours, as we sat in our car to avoid the rain and lightning, the flames finally were reduced. Left behind was a disaster. Our safe beautiful home was in ashes.

At this point, the fire chief approached our car and explained the presumed cause of the fire and the extent of the damage. Apparently, the spray foam in our attic spread the fire throughout that attic rapidly and the majority of the home was destroyed. They were able to put out the flames, but the damage to the ceiling and the drywall was extensive from a combination of the fire, the toxic fumes of the smoke, and the water necessary to put it out.

As I was barefoot and shirtless (dressed in only a pair of pants that I was able to slip on at the last second), the fire chief offered me his boots and his jacket. We then walked through the house together, and I was aghast at the destruction that had occurred in such a short time. Every single inch of the home was covered in heavy soot, so much so that you couldn't even see the colors of our furniture, walls, or the floors. The ceiling had been busted out in multiple places. Water was literally gushing through the ceiling from the second floor to the first, and we were wading through two to four inches of dirty water that had flooded the entire ground floor.

Despite the devastation, I was now able to see what the firefighters had been doing and why it took so much time. I was moved by their conscientiousness and skill. They had painstakingly laid tarp over all of our countertops in an attempt to protect our valuables. Though they were forced to break out the ceiling and flood the home with water, they rescued our family pictures off of the wall and put them in a room where there was less damage in an effort to save them.

How in the world could they be so considerate about these small things while they were literally battling a blaze that could've taken their lives? Those twenty-five brave souls had rushed into a burning home with zero visibility at risk of death for a family of strangers. I marveled at that thought.

As a physician, I have devoted my life to helping others, at times saving lives. But when you're the *recipient* of that kind of diligence and care, it really strikes you to the core. They were willing to make the ultimate sacrifice for us.

That stormy night, amazingly, nobody was injured. As I reflect on life, I am amazed about how God has always been there for us and for others. Many times, it's easy to get lost in the trials and disappointments of life and to question where God is when we most need him, but when I look back at everything that has happened to us, all I see is God's presence.

As I see it now, God was there throughout my life for every obstacle I faced, equipping me with patience, perseverance, and strength of character.

God was there when he moved the orthopaedic chairman out of the way so that I could be accepted into the orthopaedic department at Wilford Hall.

God was there every time I fell asleep at the wheel before I realized I had sleep apnea, protecting me from hurting myself or others.

God was there when he introduced me to LeAnn, my soulmate, the mother of our children, and the center of our home. It was LeAnn who was ultimately my business savior too, as it was her attention to detail that would protect me from multiple vultures who saw me as prey.

God was also there when my mentor from medical school became a Mayo Clinic spine surgeon. He paved the way for me to be accepted as the only spine fellow in the country, an action based on my performance and character, not on the labels a few of my Air Force colleagues tried to place on me.

God was there protecting me during my deployment from doubling my stay because the local commander disregarded what my chairman back home recommended.

And during many of the events described in this book, God was right there protecting me from every unjust investigation, allegation, and betrayal.

Looking back, LeAnn and I often joke about how stupid we must be for the many pitfalls we've experienced and the number of crooks we were fooled by. However, the truth is that many of them were crafty, almost genius-like in their devious ability to swindle others, but God was there to help us.

During our legal trials, God was there leading us to Eric and Mike, who ensured our victories in court and protection from false accusations. God also led us to Rod and to others who really stood up for me when my character was being called into question.

In short, God has been there for *every* part of my life, and has seen me through every challenge in it.

He was there when our friend found the box of all of my design work, invoices, and consulting work with Allure, proving I earned every dollar of my consulting agreement payments.

God was there when we found Ava, convincing her biological mother to allow us to adopt her instead of terminating the pregnancy.

And on the night of the fire, God was there giving LeAnn and me discernment to not leave and to move my smaller children into my bedroom. In fact, the lightning struck right above Ava's room and would have affected her first. God was there even in Caden's disobedience in staying in his bedroom. It was Caden who heard the lightning strike and alerted us of the fire because he had the wherewithal to understand the meaning of the billowing smoke. His quick reactions potentially saved our lives; he was one of the heroes of the night.

And God was there leading each and every one of those firefighters toward the decision to become firefighters, which ultimately led to their saving our home.

Our home is pretty much destroyed, but it is salvageable, even though it will take about two years to fix. Material things can be replaced, whereas our lives cannot be. So we are filled with gratitude only, not in the least discouraged by what happened and knowing that we have the love and support of God behind us.

It all happens for a reason. I can see that my life has been a series of obstacles and challenges. But through all of it, thanks to God, I have overcome them all. So, I thank God for every one of my trials because they have strengthened my faith and ultimately my character.

Chapter Nineteen

Pawns and Cons

Never did I expect medicine to be so cutthroat. I knew training could be grueling, mentors could be tyrannical, and the life of a doctor was not a walk in the park. What I wasn't prepared for was just how mercenary the field is. I didn't expect to become a target for so many corrupt businessmen with a financial interest in and control over what I did. I think most physicians enter medicine to truly make a difference, and we expect everyone else in medicine to be like-minded. That couldn't be further from the truth. Not only are we seen as pawns to the financial powers that control medicine, from government to commercial carriers, but also we are surrounded by con men who have been given control over the business of medicine. Physicians are held to an unreasonable standard—one to which practitioners of no other profession that I know of are held.

As doctors and businessmen, we have to make a profit to support our families, businesses, and employees. And that's becoming more and more difficult to do. The skewed system has made it *illegal* for a physician or a physician group to be more than a 40-percent owner of any business entity outside their clinics (with rare exceptions i.e., an ambulatory surgery center) that delivers care to insurance- or government-based patients. When it comes to government-funded insurance carriers, doctors can have *a* financial investment for gain from a business entity outside their clinics only in very highly regulated circumstances. Insurance companies have total control over which care is delivered, and they determine how much to pay for it. I often wonder: *In which other business does the client dictate the cost of services?* I can't think of one. And in which other business is it illegal to own the entities or to split the fees when a client is referred for services?

After all, there are multiple industries in which sharing fees or costs is standard, but doctors will go to jail for doing just that.

As a result, although we absorb the responsibility of the patient's outcome, physicians are not able to make final determinations about the services delivered nor the cost of care provided for patients. They can't even set their own prices when it comes to insurance contracts. We are paid by codes for services and surgeries, which have nothing to do with training nor outcomes. If you cut corners and work fast, you are rewarded. If you are meticulous, conscientious, and deliberate, you are penalized.

To sum it up: As insurance reimbursements continue to decline, doctors find themselves working harder, making less, and struggling to cover the costs of their medical practice. And it's impossible to make up the lost money.

Would you believe that doctors only make 10 percent of the total profit in healthcare while 90 percent goes to the businesses delivering healthcare services?

When it comes to risk for the outcomes in patient care, insurance companies assume minimal risk. Physicians bear *total* responsibility for patient outcomes. This means that the doctors—who take all the risks, do most of the work, have the most education and training, provide all of the follow-up care, and carry the responsibility for the outcomes—are making a very small fraction of the profits in medicine.

The current laws make it nearly impossible for doctors to be properly involved with the business of medicine. The crux of the problem is the many unfair laws alluded to earlier, which unreasonably limit our ability to have a voice—much less control—in what care is rendered to our patients. One of the biggest issues is the Physician Self-Referral law, commonly referred to as the Stark law, which prohibits physicians from referring patients to receive "designated health services" payable by Medicare or Medicaid from entities with which the physician or an immediate family member has a financial relationship. The law also includes Anti-Kickback legislation, which applies to all commercial (non-government) carriers.

These Anti-Kickback laws are written to "prevent unethical monetary remuneration for care." Do I think that there are unethical and unscrupulous surgeons? Of course—there are a few. But the vast majority of the ones I know, even ones who aren't great technicians, went into medicine for the right reasons.

These regulations assume physicians to be the only potentially unethical people in the equation and have been creatively used to hamstring physicians' ability to be entrepreneurial and to even make a profit.

Doctors are left absorbing massive costs to run practices that generate enormous profits for those companies. And those physicians receive no financial assistance in the cost to "capture" patients, gain their trust, and run their practices. It literally makes no sense. These rules need to be revised. It will ensure better patient care and happier physicians delivering it.

As things stand today, the venues that we refer patients to for surgery (i.e., the hospitals) do not contribute a cent to marketing for patients. If doctors receive anything of value, they go to jail. In short, the bureaucratic system and government is essentially controlling everything—the money, the access, the reimbursements.. you name it.

The financial strain is causing doctors to close their practices in ever-increasing numbers and take jobs at hospitals or other entities. At the end of 2020, 70 percent of physicians reported being employed by hospitals or corporations ("employed" physicians, as opposed to self-employed independent practitioners)—a steep acceleration from years past. In 2019, the number of employed physicians was just 46.9 percent. These arrangements often lure physicians in with hefty first-year guarantees and lofty signing bonuses. However, the arrangement shifts dramatically the second year, when physicians are held to performance standards that leave the majority of them feeling oppressed and overworked. Additionally, these physicians are now the asset of the corporate entity and are prohibited from referring patients to outside entities (i.e., labs, imaging facilities, or ambulatory surgical hospitals.) What happened to the Corporate Practice of Medicine Doctrine prohibiting corporate influence over physicians' delivery of care?

Even more concerning is the statistic that on a scale of 1 to 5 (with 5 being the most miserable) on the Physician Misery Index, employed physicians average a score of 4 out of 5! In a 2018 survey by Geneia, 89 percent of physicians reported that the current regulation of healthcare has changed the practice of medicine for the worse. Eighty-six percent of physicians agree that the heightened administrative burden and the demands of the business side of healthcare have diminished their joy in practicing medicine.

Although there is strong rhetoric that independent physicians who invest in hospitals, urgent care facilities, ancillary services, and cardiac cath labs—for example—are "greedy" and driving up the cost of healthcare, the truth is these facilities charge less for their services than hospitals delivering the same care. That's the reason hospitals are able to offer higher salaries to their employed physicians in the first place. They charge far more for physician services and the ancillary services they provide. Why is it, then, that physicians are often blamed for increasing costs in healthcare? Independent physicians are paid significantly less for their efforts and have the financial weight of massive practice overhead to cover while physician reimbursements are being steadily cut.

We are thus living in a climate of industry- and government-controlled medicine in which doctors are prohibited from or persecuted for having ownership of the business related to the delivery of care, except in our own practices. Nor can we establish a joint marketing agreement with a hospital without facing the possibility of losing our medical licenses, being federally indicted, or even imprisoned under laws that were initially intended for mafia crime lords!

These Anti-Kickback and Stark regulations have got to be revised or even *repealed*. Isn't it onerous enough that doctors face multiple tiers of restrictions in addition to the heavy responsibility for our patients' well-being? We face the continuous scrutiny of the hospital medical review committees and state and national boards—not to mention the looming threat of a medical-board complaint or the always-present danger of a lawsuit lodged by a disgruntled or money-driven patient.

All these threats, limitations, and risks for physicians are potential career-enders and—at the least—sources of incredible stress and frustration.

While physician practices were reeling from the financial effects of COVID, the top ten highest-earning CEOs of healthcare companies *each* took home more than $75 million in compensation in 2020.

COMPANY	CEO	COMPENSATION *(actual realized stock gains)*
Masimo	Joe Kiani	$210,455,014
Regeneron Pharmaceuticals	Leonard Schleifer	$174,350,089
Amedisys	Paul Kusserow	$106,123,277
IQVIA	Ari Bousbib	$93,851,775
Thermo Fisher Scientific	Marc Casper	$90,764,726
HCA Healthcare	Samuel Hazen	$83,588,767
Edwards Lifesciences	Michael Mussallem	$83,571,177
R1 RCM	Joseph Flanagan	$81,702,706
Cigna	David Cordani	$78,950,615

Many healthcare executives saw massive pay increases while physicians saw deep cuts of nearly 10 percent, triggering the president of the American Medical Association to state the rule was "a reminder of the financial peril facing physician practices at the end of the year." These cuts are commonplace in medicine.

Meanwhile, physician reimbursements are steeply declining. In fact, if you look at the reimbursements that we make today versus what doctors made for the same services in the late nineties, it is far less. Yet our rents go up by 3 percent to 5 percent every year—not to mention the increases in staff salaries and supply costs. Inflation alone is 2–3 percent per year all while physician reimbursements are constantly being decreased! It's unsustainable.

In order to avoid drowning in overhead, some surgeons feel pressured to treat more patients than they really should. This decline has led to more expedient, but not necessarily better, care. Ultimately, the result is worse outcomes—which leads to what? Increases in costs for revision surgeries, prescriptions for chronic-pain medication, and lifelong therapy and medical care. It is not good for anyone. Doctors who refuse to give in to the pressures to see a massive volume of patients to survive financially—spending mere minutes with them in clinic or flying through surgical procedures—either must join a hospital system, go into academic medicine, or seek ways to improve the delivery of care and their income (i.e., become entrepreneurial).

Ultimately, it's the insurance companies who are fostering an atmosphere in which doctors are forced to turn their practices into an assembly line with sloppier outcomes. Lower reimbursements lead some doctors to becoming more income-focused than outcome-focused. Peer-to-peer reviews limit physicians' ability to render appropriate treatment to their patients while still absorbing the responsibility for their health. The fact that insurance companies use this process to essentially practice medicine should be a concern for everyone. Limited reimbursement, denials of treatment, and clawing back of revenue all lead to increased profit for insurance carriers at the expense of the patient and financial detriment of the treating physician. No wonder doctors are looking to invest in businesses related to medicine in an effort to generate more income. The problem is that many of those arrangements violate current Anti-Kickback laws, or are created to make the businessmen money while making the doctors their worker bees.

In short, the insurance companies should not be able to determine what fees doctors are being paid. I believe it is imperative that we be able to dictate what our services are worth and not have that value determined by the very people responsible for the payments. What incentives do the insurance carriers have to pay what physician services are really worth or to deliver the best care for patients? There are none.

Doctors have to come together to actively demand better treatment and reimbursements. We're so busy complaining and working that we've done nothing to stop the insanity. Moreover, I believe there should be no in-network system at all—certainly not for specialty care. Patients deserve the best doctor: period. They deserve the right to choose their doctors based on reputation, training, and outcomes—not lists of "in-network" physicians.

Additionally, the restriction on doctors owning hospitals does nothing to improve cost or patient outcomes. That said, the Affordable Care Act did some very positive things. As a provider for patients with chronic back and/or neck pain, I was relieved when pre-existing conditions were covered by Obamacare. After all, so many patients suffering from conditions that existed before they obtained healthcare insurance were being denied care. That left a lot of people struggling to make it without appropriate medical attention. I also agreed with Obamacare making medical insurance available everyone, regardless of their income or employment situation.

When President Trump took office, I was hopeful that the unfair limitation on physician ownership of hospitals would be repealed. I was also encouraged by many of the changes

President Trump was proposing to improve the conditions of healthcare across America. One thing about the Affordable Care Act quickly became clear to me: The requirement to cover everyone came with a hefty price for many. Patients noticed dramatic increases in their insurance premiums across the board. Patient after patient complained about these increases in addition to increased deductibles and—worse yet—increased denials of coverage for requested treatments and surgeries. The insurance carriers seemed to be covering the additional patients by increasing the costs to patients who were already covered. The result was that many patients changed insurance policies or carriers for a cheaper alternative. Patients who had out-of-network coverage or PPO plans converted to in-network-only coverage and HMO plans with lower premiums and deductibles. Patients married to military members who had insurance through their employers dropped their civilian coverage, opting to be covered solely by their spouse's policy.

Peer-to-peer reviews increased dramatically. Procedures and surgeries were being restricted and denied more aggressively. Someone has to cover the cost of the additional coverage, and the carriers appear to be passing that cost off to their clients or denying more care to make up for their lost profits.

Politics aside, doctors just want someone who understands their plight and someone who helps them deliver better care for their patients. I was optimistic when the Trump administration eliminated the financial penalty for choosing not to obtain insurance coverage and pushed for competition amongst insurance carriers to lower the cost of premiums. I also agreed that companies should be allowed to pool together to decrease cost and that employees should have the option of choosing their own carrier with their employers covering the cost. Trump also encouraged tax-free medical savings plans—an excellent alternative to insurance that leaves all the control in the patients' hands. His administration also sought to decrease health insurance taxes, increase cost transparency of hospitals, and eliminate surprise billing. President Trump also made it an official United States government policy to cover pre-existing conditions and passed many reforms to decrease drug pricing. I was hopeful these changes would lead to a dramatic improvement in the cost and delivery of care and possibly increased freedom and control for physicians.

However, even these changes are a fraction of what needs to transpire to truly improve the situation for doctors and patients. The solution begins with revisiting the restrictions on entrepreneurship by physicians in the Anti-Kickback and Stark regulations. Even Pete Stark, the author of the law, says he favored repealing the law as it currently exists. It has morphed into a law of complexities and penalties that far exceed the law's original design.

I also believe doctors should be able to organize and collectively bargain for higher reimbursement from insurance carriers—and even with hospitals—to share in the massive profits they generate by bringing their patients to the facility. When professional athletes, entertainers, and fighters began to demand they receive a percentage of the profits from their efforts, they saw a dramatic increase in their incomes. It's about time for doctors to do the same.

As things stand, it's truly impossible for doctors to practice medicine the way they would want to. Once a physician is compelled to see more patients than is prudent, the quality of care declines. Add the additional volume of patients being seen to the insurmountable paperwork and documentation required of nurses, mid-levels, and physicians; and the burden becomes too heavy a weight to bear for many.

Is it any wonder that an ever-increasing number of quality students are choosing *not* to enter the field of medicine? The result of all this is that the quality of medical care in America will continue to decline. In fact, the American Association of Medical Colleges recently estimated that the U.S. could be short 37,800 to 124,000 doctors by 2034.

Especially while these regulations exist, these preposterous obstacles that physicians face must be brought to light so that physicians are able to steer clear of the pitfalls that we face on the business side of medicine. It's vital for physicians to understand the laws that exist, so they don't inadvertently violate them. But ultimately, these laws need to be re-evaluated, revised, or repealed altogether.

As if compliance with the laws and practicing credible medicine wasn't enough, physicians must also be wary of the predators waiting to capitalize on their ability to generate money *for* them.

Sadly, many doctors have been relegated to mere technicians working for taskmasters who enjoy the full benefit of the financial reward of our efforts—using our conscientiousness and education to their benefit. They've left crumbs for us to battle over, turning us against each other. The fellowship amongst physicians is all but dead.

Physicians have become their own worst enemies. As a result, the powers that be continue to control us and everything we do. The only way to make this change is to finally band together like doctors of old and become a true fellowship focused on fighting for our rights and control over what and how patient care is delivered.

Similarly, patients need to demand the care they pay for. They need to demand that their employers only use an insurance carrier that allows the patient to choose their doctor and the care they deserve and need. We can only do this together. We have little left to lose, and we and our patients have everything to gain.

My personal trials have been more extreme than I would have ever imagined, certainly more than any honest physician should ever face on the business side of medicine. Yet I know that every time I was in the midst of turmoil and despair, God would either pluck me from the situation or remove the agitator altogether.

As I reflect on my life, it is very clear that God has surrounded me with angels and put a hand of protection over me and my family despite the constant stream of attacks I have experienced.

In the end, like all trials, I used them to strengthen me and to improve my understanding of my place in the world. They made me more grateful for all that I had been given. None of the adversities of life deterred me. Conversely, whatever challenges I encountered actually encouraged and spurred me on to work *harder*, to draw closer to God, and to my family.

I learned to appreciate my wife for everything she has been in my life—my true love, my defender, the object of my affection, and the one person who grounds me. I know for sure that, without LeAnn's diligence, organization, foresight, and intuition, I would have had a difficult time defending myself from the many false allegations that came my way. Physically, I could protect her from many things, but she protected me from attacks that required her special strengths. As I've mentioned, she is an organizational genius and kept detailed records that proved every allegation to be untrue, protecting me from possible destruction. Indeed, Lord knows, without her, there's a chance that I would have been indicted and possibly even convicted for crimes I never committed. For that grace, I am eternally grateful.

As a result of all our troubles, our relationship has actually strengthened. Together we knew that even if the world was against us, God had our back—and we had each other's.

I also found sanctity in my family and in my four children. When I arrive home each day, their beautiful smiles and careless laughter always lighten my spirit. So, I pour myself into family time, recognizing the true blessings they are in my life. Without them, where would I be mentally or physically? I thank God every day for each and every one of my children and for their loving mother.

In addition, I must give eternal thanks to my mother and in-laws who were all there for me every night, sometimes as late as 11:00 p.m., helping to take care of me when my family moved to Houston. No matter what was happening, they always offered an empathetic ear and a warm meal ready for me when I arrived home late. Their kindness sustained me, as did my faith.

I have also had some very faithful friends who proved themselves loyal when so many others had turned their backs on me. They came to my defense, putting themselves and their own relationships on the line to prove my innocence.

Many times, I would turn to the Bible and read Matthew, Romans, and Psalms, just to ease my spirit. And God was always there to guide me, to uplift me, and to give me strength to persevere.

As I see it now, I have dedicated my life to my family and to my patients, and for that reason, my life has been fulfilling in every way. I would add that my mental focus and sense of inner calm are immeasurably enhanced by my physical strength and focus on nutrition, health, and exercise. So, my life is a combination of faith and focus, and I have overcome every trial, every battle I have faced thus far.

But despite all the supports in place, with the love of God, my family, and self-care, there is no magic formula to happiness. Life is not easy for any of us. We all face our own trials and challenging circumstances. That's inevitable, but it's how we prepare for, face, and respond to those battles that counts. The way we behave dictates how we will be remembered and what kind of representative we were of God.

Sometimes in times of trial, we react badly and our relationships suffer. How many marriages have not survived such crises? Yet LeAnn and I believe that a relationship built on faith should be strengthened by trials, not weakened by them. In fact, without that faith, few couples could have survived the difficult trials that we faced.

True, on our own, our flesh is too weak, and our minds are too feeble to battle many of the challenges we face as humans, but with Jesus in the center of our lives, we have someone who's fighting for us, who gives us guidance, motivation, mental peace, strength, and, ultimately, protection from the sins of the world.

I truly believe my life is clear evidence of that. Every one of my successes in life, including my surgical successes, comes from the fact that I am faithfully devoted to living a Christ-like life.

I am far from perfect, but my desire is to be a good representative, a good human, to take care of my fellow man, to be an example of strength and faithful perseverance to those around me, especially my children. As Nelson Mandela so aptly stated, "I never lose. I either win or I learn." You have to adapt and overcome, and you also have to have an indomitable spirit.

In the end, as I learned, family is everything. As we tell our children, faith is what sets the foundation. Be each other's cheerleaders and let trials strengthen your relationships, not divide or tear them apart.

I always tell them to surround themselves with a small circle of genuine friends and to be very wary of anyone who compliments them incessantly, paints a grand picture of the future, and makes lofty promises. In our case, although we tried to give people the benefit of the doubt, we've been burned so often that we realized we can truly only trust God, each other, and few others.

As our kids have seen, the trials we went through taught us how to be self-reliant and how to build our lives with our own efforts. Though we were often betrayed and cheated, it was those experiences that forced us how to grow and succeed on our own. As it says in *Romans 5:3–5*—"*...but we also glory in our sufferings, because we know that suffering produces perseverance; perseverance, character; and character, hope. And hope does not put us to shame, because God's love has been poured out into our hearts through the Holy Spirit, who has been given to us.*"

Our troubles allowed our kids to see us fail and come back again, multiple times, due to sheer will power, faith, and grit. They even saw how being too generous can hurt you. Hopefully, our difficulties will give them the protective awareness they need to avoid similar pitfalls in their own future businesses and how to lean on God when they fail despite their best efforts.

You may recall my story earlier about the time the chairman of orthopaedics told me, "You must lead a good life, because it seems that God is always there to protect you."

Thinking of what he said reminds me of the story of Daniel, who was cast into the lion's den after disobeying a law prohibiting praying to anyone other than the king. When Daniel was thrown into that den and forced to spend the night there, the king found him unharmed the next morning.

Daniel explained, "God sent an angel to close the mouths of the lions because I was found blameless before him." I believe God did the same for me, each and every time I was cast into the pit, surrounded by the lions in my life. Though threatened by predators, I emerged unharmed every time. For that, I am eternally grateful.

Most of all, as I've learned from Him, the key to happiness is to live a life of integrity, faith, and truth. In the end, the truth will set you free. It did for us.

John 8:31–32—"So Jesus said to the Jews who had believed in him, 'If you abide in my word, you are truly my disciples, and you will know the truth, and the truth will set you free.'"

END

Acknowledgments

This book is, at its core, all about God's love and protection in my life despite the many trials I experienced. I could not have written it nor gotten through it all, without my strong faith and the people who are dearest to me.

First and foremost, no words suffice for my wonderful wife of twenty-two years, LeAnn. She is the heart and soul of our family—my best friend, life partner, the most attentive mother imaginable, the true source of my happiness.

I sometimes jokingly refer to her as a "trophy" wife, *not* because of her beauty, which is indisputable. It's because of her *mind*. As you read, she is not the stereotypical "doctor's wife," but instead, the brains behind the operations of both our businesses and medical practice.

Her steadfastness, strength, insight, and intuition have protected us all, and my life would be incomplete without her.

I also must thank our four incredible children—Alexa, Colton, Caden, and Ava—each uniquely talented and special. On a daily basis, they motivate and inspire me to be a better dad and a better person. They comprise my entire world.

Special thanks to my mother, the epitome of style and grace, who raised me to be a gentleman. From an early age, she taught me to respect myself and others. From her, I also learned to be proud of my heritage and to appreciate the opportunities made possible as an American. Rain or shine, she has always been there for our family, ready with motherly medical advice, a meal, and a warm smile! She's the ultimate mom.

I want to equally thank my father for instilling in me such a strong worth ethic—a drive for perfection, academic excellence, and the value of serving others. From him, I learned never to give up no matter what the circumstance. Though he is in Heaven now, he is still very much with us all.

A special debt of gratitude to my mother-in-law and father-in-law, Carol and Jack Bergerud, who were always there for me late after work with a feast fit for a king. They have showered me with love and have been amazing grandparents to my children.

I also have to thank my big brother, Bryan, for always being my biggest cheerleader and protector growing up. We had many great adventures I'll never forget, and he always made me feel like part of his crew even though I was the "little" brother.

I want to thank my little brother, Michael, nine years younger than me. Because of him, I learned how to care for a baby, how to be a good role model, and what it was like to have someone younger look up to me. My only regret is that we were so far apart in age that we had little time together during his formative years.

I also want to acknowledge my brother-in-law, John Bergerud, who has been there for us any and every time we needed anything. He spends countless hours promoting our practice and my surgeries on the Internet and social media, making it possible to highlight what we do for the masses.

Finally, I want to thank my extended family in the Philippines and Spain, the Centeneras and Ceas, for always throwing a celebration every time we visited. They made us feel proud to be part of the family and made it obvious we were special to them.

In the creation of this book, LeAnn has been patiently involved every step of the way, contributing her vivid memories, insight, and skills as a researcher, helping me sift through years of our memorabilia, records, and correspondence.

As far as the actual production of this book is concerned, I want to thank my amazing collaborator, best-selling author Glenn Plaskin, who helped me formulate a coherent account of my life. Glenn was invaluable as a source of insight and literary genius. He worked with me to recount many years of complicated twists and turns that would have confused anyone. I am grateful for his patience and diligence, but mostly for his talent and for the friendship we developed while writing this book together.

I also want to thank our publisher at Amplify Books, who believed in our story and brought it to the world. Naren Aryal and his team meticulously edited, designed, guided, and produced the book in your hand. In particular, our editor, Rebecca Andersen, who provided her tremendous talent in organizing the content and provided insight that has only made the book's message clearer and more succinct. I also give thanks to Brandon Coward and the publicity and marketing team who have worked so hard to make this book a success.

More gratitude on a personal note:

We owe a life-long debt to our nanny, Ashley, who is like a daughter to us. Over the years, she has become LeAnn's executive assistant, and she has tirelessly helped LeAnn collect and organize all the files we needed through the years no matter what the challenge, legal and otherwise.

As far as professional associations go, I want to acknowledge the many amazing mentors in medicine and surgery who have instilled in me the knowledge and skills necessary to do what I do best. Some who impacted me most were Dr. Carlos Pestana, dean of my medical school; Dr. Jose Trabal, my ob-gyn professor who taught me to present "eloquently"; Dr. Fred Corley, my orthopaedic surgery advisor, whose humility and work ethic inspired all budding orthopaedic surgeons at the University of Texas.

Special thanks to the unforgettable Dr. Michael Yaszemski, who has been my orthopaedic mentor since I was a medical student and whose specialty I chose to pursue. Your guidance over the years has been invaluable in everything I do and every patient I help. Dr. Ted Parsons, one of the most intelligent and gifted orthopaedic surgeons I have ever met; Dr. Bradford Currier, the brilliant spine surgeon who trained me at the Mayo Clinic, inspiring me to learn and perfect my craft as a surgeon; Dr. Paul Huddleston, another Mayo mentor, who was like the wiser older brother who always made me feel at ease, guiding me with an empathic ear and a compassionate response.

Like me, my cosmetic surgery mentor, Dr. Wilbur Hah, was an outside-the-box thinker. He took me on as a fellow, even though he was trying to slow down his practice at the time. As the president of the American Board of Cosmetic Surgery, he convinced the entire board to accept me as a fellow, although they had never trained an orthopaedic surgeon and weren't sure if I would be a good fit. I want to thank him for taking a chance and for training me. He has continued to be a resource of knowledge and encouragement for me in my cosmetic surgery practice. He is a gracious and conscientious mentor to whom I will always be grateful.

I also want to also acknowledge the people in the OR who support what I do every single day to improve the lives of our patients: Dr. Bertrand Brown, Dr. Andy Bowser, Dr. Davinder Bhatia, Dr. JC Walkes, Glenn Flojo, Rod Batson, John Wesley, Brian Retz, Joe Nuno, Jay and Lou Castaneda, Holly McClure, and Reggie Naylor. I'll will never forget the contributions of Lisa Cerda, Mizeny Romo, Angie O'Neill, Jeff Buysse, and Rebecca Moron, all of whom took care of my patients during my years at Innova and Victory Hospitals.

I thank all the talented anesthesiologists, CRNAs, nurses, and scrub technicians I have met in my career who were equally devoted to delivering amazing care to patients. Much deserving of gratitude is my current team in San Antonio and Houston—Dr. Thomson, Dr. Pinsky, Damon Tanous, Josh Wheat, Matt Kelly, Rob Garza, and Josh Bates, Jamie Pirkle, Becca Arrison, and Janene McKnight, and all the amazing preop, PACU, and floor nurses at First Colony (my Houston crew) as well as Cheri Whitaker, Marisa Pacheco, and Azmita Mohammed, and the amazing preop, PACU, and floor nurses at the BOH (my SA crew), to name the few who help me most often.

In terms of my military career, I want to thank all my colleagues in the Air Force who believed in me, who protected me, and who stood by me when the hornets were swarming. I also want to thank every patient I was honored to care for when they were injured serving our country.

I want to thank Mark Weitz, our outstanding clinic attorney, for his years of dedication to protecting the practice. I want to extend heartfelt gratitude to his brother Tim Weitz, the previous general counsel to the Texas Medical Board, who has skillfully guided me and protected my interests over the years. His legal skill and professionalism are second to none.

I'm also thankful to Ron Johnson, my bankruptcy attorney, for doing everything he could to protect and aid me when I needed it most. Ron really believed in me and became close to me and LeAnn through this process. He fought hard for our victory and to prove our case despite battling stage 4 cancer through it all. He was a true warrior and defender of truth. Ron, sadly, passed away prior to the release of this book. I pray he knows how much his friendship and efforts were appreciated.

Lenny Vitullo, our steadfast attorney, who inspired me with his strong sense of justice, going after the money that was stolen from LeAnn's family trust. Lenny is definitely one of the good guys, and we are indebted to him for his skill and integrity.

Eric Taube, the masterful lawyer who single-handedly defended me, LeAnn, and her family trust against a large team of very well-funded and vicious adversaries and a biased judge. We could not have won so many victories in court without him, I am sure. I am confident he is one of the most masterful bankruptcy attorneys in the country.

To my close friends Glenn Flojo and Rod Batson, who also came to my defense, proving my innocence and defending my name, I thank God for your honesty and friendship.

A special debt of gratitude to Michael McCrum, our defense attorney, a man of great integrity who provided such an intelligent and careful approach to clearing my name from false allegations.

Mike's talent, honesty, faith, and dedication to justice have imprinted on both me and LeAnn for a lifetime.

Sincere thanks to our healthcare attorney, who has ensured every single contract and agreement was compliant and safe over my entire career. He has been a consistent advisor over many years and has been an invaluable guide in our medical investments. He has truly been a Godsend for us.

I also want to thank our current practice administrator, Liz Marshall-Trevino, for operating an efficient and dignified practice. Special thanks to our physical therapist, Marcus Trejo, our pain specialists, Dr. Mike Mckee and Dr. Anjali Jain, as well as our PAs—Paul Chen, and Mary Vuong, who take such diligent care of our preoperative and postoperative patients and to Brent Eaton, FNP, for enthusiastically helping me in the operating room, the hospital, and clinic. I want to also acknowledge Dr. Stanley Jones, an amazing surgeon and person, who has entrusted me with the surgical care of his Houston patients; my entire SA and Houston clinic staff in both spine and cosmetic surgery. Also, to the amazing doctors who follow and care for my patients postoperatively and the referring doctors who trust me with the surgical care of their patients—a heartfelt thank you. I couldn't do what I do without all of you.

I want to thank our previous CEO, Linda D'Spain, for "cleaning house," divesting us of all those who were dragging the practice down and enhancing our operation with ease. She and her husband, Ron, have become dear friends and I am forever thankful to them for being there for my family.

Thank you to our longtime accountant, Bert Gonzalez, of the Gonzalez Group, for making sure our financial records are always meticulous and accurate.

Outside the hospital and office, I have to acknowledge my brothers-in-Christ, dear friends Nico and Davida LaHood and Jorge and Stephanie Araujo, who were always there with sage biblical advice and much-needed prayers during our most difficult times. Their friendship is a true example of "iron sharpening iron."

Cheers also to Mark and Heather Magarian, who stayed true friends to us through it all, with Mark providing an empathic ear and invaluable investment advice.

I also want to acknowledge Anita and Jerry Caballero, who have been our close friends for many years. Not only do they help manage our skincare and nutrition lines, but they have also helped us to coordinate and celebrate many special occasions, including birthdays, anniversaries, and charity events. They have been an invaluable source of friendship and support over the years.

I want to thank all my former classmates and teachers from Clark Air Base and East Central High School who have continued to send me messages of support and praise over the years. I love you all and appreciate having you in my past and current life.

Special thanks to my college roommate, Scott Moore, and his lovely wife, Tammy, who are our most constant and genuine friends, rare gems in this world.

Not least, since home is where the heart is, I also want to thank my hometown of San Antonio, which embraced me when I returned from a nearly eight-year overseas assignment. I have come to love that community and the many people who have shown faith in me and my practice and business pursuits. I am also grateful to the vibrant and diverse city of Houston, which has welcomed me and my family warmly in recent years. A special debt of gratitude goes out to the firefighters of the Spring, Klein, and Woodlands Fire Departments for coming to our aid that fateful night of the fire.

Finally, and most importantly, I want to thank God, and my Lord, Jesus, the sole source of my blessings in this life. He is my guiding light, my true north, my reason for living. I strive to model a Christ-like life and make a true difference in the world. On a daily basis, as I watch my children grow up, I pray for His continued guidance and protection.

As you saw, my journey has been one of trials and triumph—with God squarely in the middle of it. As it says in Romans 8:31, "If God is for us, who can be against us?"

As it turned out, quite a few!

Source Material

American Medical Association. "Wake Up to Financial Peril Facing Medicare Payment System." July 21, 2021. https://www.ama-assn.org/press-center/press-releases/ama-wake-financial-peril-facing-medicare-payment-system.

Association of American Medical Colleges. "AAMC Report Reinforces Mounting Physician Shortage." June 11, 2021. https://www.aamc.org/news-insights/press-releases/aamc-report-reinforces-mounting-physician-shortage.

Brown, Alyson. "Forest Park: Key Takeaways for Health Care Professionals and Their Lawyers." Clouse Brown PLLC. May 7, 2019. https://clousebrown.com/forest-park-trial-takeaways/.

Carlson, Joe. "Pete Stark: Repeal the Stark Law." Modern Healthcare. August 2, 2013. https://www.modernhealthcare.com/article/20130802/BLOG/308029995/pete-stark-repeal-the-stark-law

"Doctors Are Pawns of Health Care System." KevinMD. November 9, 2018. https://www.kevinmd.com/blog/2018/11/doctors-are-pawns-of-the-health-care-system.html.

Dyrda, Laura. "70% of Physicians Are Now Employed by Hospitals or Corporations." Becker's ASC Review. July 1, 2021. https://www.beckersasc.com/asc-transactions-and-valuation-issues/70-of-physicians-are-now-employed-by-hospitals-or-corporations.html.

Fisher, Ken. "Corporate Medicine Uses Doctors as Pawns." Medical Economics. May 27, 2017. https://www.medicaleconomics.com/view/corporate-medicine-use-doctors-pawns.

Frieden, Joyce. "Final Physician Fee Schedule Rule Includes a Nearly 4% Payment Cut." Medpage Today. November 3, 2021. https://www.medpagetoday.com/practicemanagement/reimbursement/95421.

Geneia. "Physician Misery Index Increases to Nearly 4 Out Of 5." Press release. October 30, 2018. https://www.geneia.com/resources/news/press-releases/2018/October/Physician-Misery-Index-increases-to-nearly-4-out-of-5.

Gordon, Mara. "Novelist Doctor Skewers Corporate Medicine In 'Man's 4th Best Hospital.'" NPR. November 13, 2019. https://www.npr.org/sections/health-shots/2019/11/13/777688384/novelist-doctor-skewers-corporate-medicine-inmans-4th-best-hospital.

Herman, Bob. "Health Care Executive Pay Soars during Pandemic." Axios. June 14, 2021. https://www.axios.com/health-care-ceo-pay-2020-pandemic-fb585a6c-dd1d-4a20-8561-44a6bac6d39d.html.

Hones, Jeffrey M., and RJ Reinhart. "Americans Remain Dissatisfied With Healthcare Costs." Gallup. November 28, 2018. https://news.gallup.com/poll/245054/americans-remain-dissatisfied-health-care-costs.aspx.

"Impact of Future Medicare Cuts on Physician Reimbursement." Revcycle Intelligence. August 24, 2021. https://revcycleintelligence.com/news/impact-of-future-medicare-cuts-on-physician-reimbursement.

Jauhar, Sandeep. "Why Doctors Are Sick of Their Profession." *Wall Street Journal*. August 29, 2014. https://online.wsj.com/articles/the-u-s-s-ailing-medical-system-a-doctors-perspective-1409325361.

Kaplan, Robert S., and Michael E. Porter. "The Big Idea: How to Solve the Cost Crisis in Health Care." *Harvard Business Review*. September 2011. https://hbr.org/2011/09/how-to-solve-the-cost-crisis-in-health-care.

Krause, Kevin. "These Guys Smuggled Medical Pot to Dallas after They'd Been Arrested for Healthcare Fraud, Feds Say." *Dallas Morning News*. July 23, 2018. https://www.dallasnews.com/news/crime/2018/07/23/these-guys-smuggled-medical-pot-to-dallas-after-they-d-been-arrested-for-health-care-fraud-feds-say/.

Lyon, Michael. "The Obama Health Plan Has Serious Threats to Medicare." Healthcare-Now!. https://www.healthcare-now.org/blog/the-obama-health-plan-has-serious-threats-to-medicare/.

Maxwell, Yael L. "Some Good News, Some Bad in Proposed 2021 CMS Reimbursement Changes." TCTMD. August 7, 2020. https://www.tctmd.com/news/new-guidance-use-diabetes-drugs-cvd-risk-reduction-acc-experts.

Morris, Seger S., and Heather Lusby. "The Physician Compensation Bubble Is Looming." American Association for Physician Leadership. January 16, 2019. https://www.physicianleaders.org/news/physician-compensation-bubble-looming.

Page, Leigh. "8 Ways That the ACA Is Affecting Doctors' Incomes." Medscape. August 15, 2013. https://www.medscape.com/viewarticle/809357.

Pollock, Jordan R., Tanner R. Bollig, Jack M. Haglin, Benjamin J. Sandefur, Douglas E. Rappaport, and Rachel A. Lindor. "Medicare Reimbursement to Physicians Decreased for Common Emergency Medicine Services from 2000 to 2020." *Annals of Emergency Medicine* 76. no. 5 (November 2020): 615-620. https://pubmed.ncbi.nlm.nih.gov/33097121/.

Probasco, Jim. "Why Do Healthcare Costs Keep Rising?" Investopedia. June 10, 2021. https://www.investopedia.com/insurance/why-do-healthcare-costs-keep-rising/.

Ramirez Jr., Domingo. "Forest Park Hospital Co-founder Sentenced in $200 million Dallas-Fort Worth Fraud Case." *Fort Worth Star-Telegram*. August 11, 2020. https://www.star-telegram.com/news/local/crime/article244878962.html.

Schulte, Fred, Elizabeth Lucas, and Kaiser Health News. "The Spinal Tap: Device Makers Have Funneled Billions to Orthopedic Surgeons Who Use Their Products." Fortune. June 17, 2021. https://fortune.com/2021/06/17/device-makers-funneled-billions-to-surgeons-products-spinefrontier/.

Trump Administration White House Archive. December 5, 2021. https://trumpwhitehouse.archives.gov/.

United States Department of Justice. The United States Attorney's Office—Western District of Texas. "14 Defendants Sentences to 74+ Years in Forest Park Healthcare Fraud." March 19, 2021. https://www.justice.gov/usao-ndtx/pr/14-defendants-sentenced-74-years-forest-park-healthcare-fraud.

United States Department of Justice. The United States Attorney's Office—Western District of Texas. "Former U.S. Army Physician Sentenced to Federal Prison for his Role in an Estimated $7.3 Million Health Care Fraud Scheme." September 25, 2015. https://www.justice.gov/usao-wdtx/pr/former-us-army-physician-sentenced-federal-prison-his-role-estimated-73-million-health.

"The War on Specialists." *Wall Street Journal*. October 6, 2009. https://www.wsj.com/articles/SB10001424052748704471504574443472658898710.